The Magic Bullet: Revolutionizing Drug Delivery

Shireen

First Printing, 2024

Table of Contents

Page

Chapter 1: Introduction

The severe nature of acute systemic toxicity is generally associated with seizure, cardiovascular and respiratory failures.[1] Limiting the drug dosage to a narrow therapeutic window is the most commonly used solution to prevent circulatory toxicity.[2] However, the therapeutic efficiency is directly related to the local concentration of the drug. The meeting point between the maximum safe drug concentration and ample therapeutic efficacy is not generally desirable. Thus, traditional molecular medicine required a new innovative perspective to address the problem of low therapeutic index.

The revolutionary ideology of drug delivery systems was first introduced in 1909.[3] The magic bullet concept introduced a balancing bridge between therapeutic effects and side effects. This foundation had been under development for years, till in the late 1950s, when Beecham developed the first functional drug delivery system.[4] Since 1950, a variety of different material compositions have become increasingly recognized as potential delivery systems. Regardless of their differences, the very final goal of any delivery system is to increase the therapeutic index of each administered pharmaceutical compound by preventing systemic toxicity and maintaining a protected drug interaction with only the diseased tissue.[5] These therapeutic tools were developed to provide the opportunity to get direct access to the target sites with reduced overall side effects.

Since their development in the 1960s, liposomes have been widely investigated because of their physicochemical, and biological advantages.[6] Liposomes are versatile drug carriers because of their morphological similarities to plasma membrane[7] and the flexibility in their formulation (i.e. they can be made from different synthetic and natural lipids).[8] In addition to being used as drug delivery vehicles, liposomes are also commonly used as a model to study cell membrane behavior.[9,10] However, in order to create biomimetic drug delivery carriers, it is often necessary to incorporate proteins in the liposome structure, either to enhance targeting efficiency or to better mimic membrane properties.[11]

Previous studies by Pamar et al.[12] and Angrand et al.[13] have shown the possibility of using detergent-mediated dialysis in order to reconstitute few proteins into the liposomes. Nevertheless, it is very difficult to incorporate proteins in the liposome structure to ensure of their proper targeting ability, and/or to use them as biomimetic models.[14] These technical difficulties have led to the search for better biomimetics including vesicles isolated directly from the live cells.

Cell-derived giant plasma membrane vesicle (GPMV) refers to an assembled cytoskeleton- and nuclear-free membrane and is obtained from chemically induced vesiculation techniques in mammalian cells.[15] GPMVs are suitable candidates for drug encapsulation and delivery that limits the potential toxicity and contains all membrane proteins.[16] Therefore, they are suitable tools for the improvement of drug delivery systems and nanoparticle-cell membrane cytotoxicity studies. My overall hypothesis is that surface engineering and chemical composition of lipid bilayer membranes controls their interactions with cells and exogenous materials. I propose the following aims:

Aim 1. Investigate the localization of functionalized liposomes to cells overexpressing VCAM1 under static and flow conditions.

Aim 2. Investigate the feasibility of using GPMVs as a drug delivery system.

Aim 3. Investigate the role of proteins and lipids in nanoparticle-cell membrane interactions.

In this dissertation, I have first functionalized liposomes using the antibodies against VCAM1 to guide and release the encapsulated therapeutics in a controlled manner to cells overexpressing this protein. Then, using GPMVs as an advanced biological membrane model, I have investigated the potential novel, core-shell drug delivery strategy. Finally, I utilized GPMVs as a biomimetic membrane to study the different mechanisms of nanoparticle-membrane interaction/cytotoxicity based on the membrane proteins function.

Surface-Functionalized Liposomes for Atherosclerosis Targeting

Liposomal delivery platforms can be used to carry a wide variety of hydrophobic and hydrophilic drugs with fewer adverse side effects, and overall drug dose reduction compared to polymeric nanoparticles.[17] The lipid bilayer structure of liposomes causes a low level of plasma membrane damages with reduced cytotoxic effects.[18] The biologically relevant composition of lipids can modulate liposomal interaction with different cells[19] and increase their molecular uptake.[20] Liposome-cell membrane fusion, liposome internalization by endocytosis (pinocytosis and phagocytosis), and receptor-mediated cellular uptake are some of the methods that can explain liposome uptake and cytoplasmic delivery.[21,22]

Circulation time in blood vessels is highly dependent on the surface and structural properties of nanoparticles and can be improved through surface modification.[23] While liposomes are rapidly removed from the circulatory system after the systemic injection, due to the action of phagocytes,[24] PEGylated liposomes have been shown to reduce phagocytosis[25] and increase the circulation time.[26] Atherosclerosis refers to the inflammatory process of plaque formation and lipid accumulation under a dysfunctional endothelium monolayer.[27,28]

Advanced atherosclerosis is the principal cause of heart attack and stroke nationally and accounts for more deaths and disability than all cancers combined.[29] There are currently many clinical trials in the process to prevent or slow the progression of atherosclerosis using different drugs. However, severe side effects have been reported following the prescription of these synthetic drugs including insulin resistance and type II diabetes.[30] Therefore, new localized therapeutic strategies are strongly needed to prevent or treat atherosclerosis. During the past two decades, peptide-functionalized delivery systems have been intensively investigated because of their ability to avoid systemic toxicity, while providing sufficient local drug concentration over the conventional dosage treatments.[31,32]

Besides, several pathological studies in the human and animal models demonstrated overexpression of VCAM1 molecules on the surface of the endothelial cells during the immunoinflammatory response in atherosclerosis.[33, 34,35,36] Multiple studies have already investigated the use of anti-VCAM1 motifs in their drug delivery cargos. In one of these delivery efforts, Sun et al. have functionalized gold nanoparticles with an atherogenic miRNA inhibitory compound and anti-VCAM1 antibody to deliver therapeutics to inflamed endothelium.[37] Also, Drs. Goetz and Malgor have performed another targeted delivery experiment that indicates VCAM1 functionalized solid particles are capable to target the atherosclerotic plaques.[34] The *in vitro* and *in vivo* targetability of anti-VCAM1 functionalized peptide amphiphiles and perfluorocarbon nanoparticles have been studied by Mlinar et al.[38] and Pan et al.[39] using the mouse models with atherosclerosis disorder.

Hemodynamic shear stress is an important factor that has to be considered in more accurate *in vitro* studies. Meanwhile, many studies have not investigated this aspect of delivery systems. Previous studies have revealed the importance of mimicking hydrodynamic conditions of blood flow on endothelial cell morphology and cytoskeletal alignment.[40] Shear stress-induced studies have shown mechanical forces alter alignment, elongation, metabolic response, and different penetration levels of nanoparticles in endothelial cells under flow versus static conditions.[41,42] To consider this aspect, I decided to use a parallel plate cell flow chamber to examine the targetability of VCAM-1 functionalized liposomes under physiologically relevant flow conditions.

In conclusion, there have been several research activities to develop an ample targeting delivery system for atherosclerosis. However, the hard and polymeric nature of their carriers caused low cellular uptake and release levels.[43] To address these shortcomings, I show in this dissertation research that soft and biodegradable lipid membranes are capable of releasing the core compounds upon their uptake in the recipient cells after getting functionalized using the suitable motifs. Also, I have investigated the liposome binding under the shear stress of blood flow to enhance the accuracy and reliability of this study.

Cell Membrane-Derived Structures for Drug Delivery

While the nanoparticle field has undergone explosive growth over the past few decades, there are still several important factors that need exploration. Developing non-invasive platforms with a high level of structural and/or functional similarity to biological membranes is highly desirable to reduce toxicity.[44] Numerous studies have been performed concerning the impact of the physicochemical properties of engineered biomimetic nanoparticles on their interaction with cells.[45,46] Nevertheless, even the newest and most cutting-edge biological nanoparticles do not provide sufficient structural, mechanical, biochemical, and biological resemblance to the cellular membrane.[46] Plasma membrane, as the initial boundary of the cell, regulates all the outer cellular interactions with exogenous particles.[47] These ordered complex assemblies include compartmentalized proteins,[48] enabling substrates to flow in and out of compartments, and activating complex biochemical reactions including signal transduction and element transmission to a receiving cell.[49]

Membrane proteins facilitate cellular trafficking,[48] cellular membrane interactions, and drug delivery via tethering the nanovesicles to specific proteins outside the cell.[50] Albeit all membrane proteins are located at the membrane, little is known about their exact location, order, orientation, and the mechanism underlying their compartmentalization.[51] Besides the fact that containing proteins in delivery platforms must be appreciable because of their increased ability in membrane biomimicry, it is also important to investigate their specific role in cellular targeting, binding and delivery processes.

Cell-derived giant plasma membrane vesicles (GPMVs) are micron-sized cell blebs, which are isolated directly from living cells by chemical induction. Although these blebs still contain parental cytoplasm, they have been shown to lack cellular (internal) organelles.[15] GPMVs offer a close approximation for the intact plasma membrane by maintaining the compositional complexity, protein positioning relative to the other membrane proteins in a fluid-mosaic pattern, as well as the physical and mechanical properties of the cellular membrane.[52] As a result, GPMVs have been widely studied and used to investigate membrane mechanical properties,[53] lipid-lipid, and lipid-protein interactions.[54]

GPMVs can also be of interest as drug delivery vehicles. Several in vitro studies have estimated the drug loading capacity of cellular membrane structure despite the absence of phagocytosis mechanism.[16,55] Saalik et al.[56] have demonstrated that small cell-penetrating peptides were internalized inside GPMVs. Yet not all studied peptides were able to penetrate inside the GPMV lumen, but only the small peptides that were already confirmed to have the ability to cross the cell membrane.[56,57] According to the research by Skinkle et al.[58], GPMVs have also been proven suitable for the permeation and loading of hydrophilic therapeutics smaller than 40 kDa through the heterogeneous pores that were formed during the rupture of vesicles from cells.

In this dissertation, I aimed to evaluate the ability of GPMVs as a core-shell structure to encapsulate nanomaterials in their core. While this is a proof-of-concept system, using particles in a core-shell structure has already been applied in therapeutic delivery applications. Creixell et al.[59] have confirmed the cancer therapeutic applications of magnetic nanoparticle heaters; iron oxide nanoparticles were shown to cause cell death mediated by intracellular magnetic hyperthermia. Similarly, silicon oxide nanoparticles were employed to passivate the progression of cancer as demonstrated by Premnath et al.[60] Therefore, it is observed that nanoparticles can be utilized for several biological applications such as in the development of biosensors, separation of molecular components, cellular MRI probes, and drug delivery.[61,62]

In this dissertation, I have evaluated a novel loading method by incubating nanoparticles with the parent cells prior to vesiculation. The lumen of GPMVs contained these drugs and nanoparticles from the cytoplasm of parental cells. Considering the fact that therapeutics can utilize both endocytosis and direct penetration mechanisms using this method, more variety of drugs and nanoparticles can gain entry to these core-shell delivering cargos.

Understanding the Function of Different Lipids and Proteins in Nanoparticle-Induced Cytotoxicity

The increasing use of nanoparticles as drug delivery tools and in consumer products has raised safety concerns regarding their potential deleterious health effects.[63] Several in-vivo studies have proved the toxic effects of nanoparticles in the brain, central nervous system, liver, spleen, and kidney of the mouse and rat models.[64,65] Moreover, several in vitro studies have shown that nanoparticles can induce cell toxicity through oxidative stress, inflammation, and inhibition of cell division.[63,66,67] Silica nanoparticles are particularly useful as a particle model for such studies.

Silica-based nanoparticles have been widely used in industrial applications for coatings, printing, and polishing. The widespread use of silica nanoparticles has also been studied as drug delivery agents, imaging probe systems, and other therapeutic purposes.[68] Kim et al. have proposed that the cellular toxicity level of silica nanoparticles is size-, dose- and cell type-dependent.[69] In vitro toxicity studies using silica nanoparticles (with mean diameters of 46-104 nm and 100-500 μg/ml concentration) revealed a significant decrease in cell viability in A549 cells after 24 hours.[66,69] However, other studies have not shown significant toxicity by these particles in A549 cells.[70,71]

The conflicting evidence from both in vitro and in vivo toxicological studies shows that further research into nanoparticle-induced cytotoxicity and their specific mechanism of action is required.[72] It has been shown that nanoparticles can freely transfer through the cell membrane using the endocytosis process to induce cytotoxicity inside the cell;[73] however, the mechanisms of toxicity to the plasma membrane itself remains ambiguous.

The plasma membrane of mammalian cells is composed of approximately 50% lipid and 50% protein by weight.[74] Over the years, numerous studies have examined the composition and behavior of membrane lipids[75] and utilized membrane models to study biophysical characteristics of the plasma membrane.[76],[77] However, these biologically relevant systems cannot mimic the exact lipid orientation and protein composition in the complex asymmetric structure of cell membranes.[78] Also, the lipid composition of plasma membrane changes over time and from one cell type to another in response to other variables including the diet or disease.[75]

Due to all the difficulties and complexities of mimicking the plasma membrane, researchers are still searching for an appropriate model to understand the mechanisms of nanotoxicity and examine nanomaterial-cell membrane interactions. GPMVs can help address many of the challeneges of nanoparticle-biomembrane interactions by providing the lipid/protein composition of the native plasma membrane without interference from endocytosis. Wang et al.[63] have reported that nanoparticles are able to penetrate the plasma membrane through a non-endocytic passive penetration method. The attachment and passive diffusion process of nanoparticles, as the leading causes of the membrane fluctuations, are critical cytotoxicity mechanisms that lead to the formation of holes and rupturing[79] or disruption of the membrane integrity.[80]

Nevertheless, natural plasma membranes are intrinsically complex and difficult to manipulate. Therefore, the function of membrane lipids and/or proteins in nanoparticle–membrane interactions are still unclear. Here, I studied the exogenously-induced toxicity using three different surface chemistries, including carboxylate, amine, and plain modified silica nanoparticles (50 nm). Taken together, the GPMV membrane model can be a valuable source in overcoming these complexities.

Chapter 2: Functionalized Liposomes for VCAM1-Targeted Drug Delivery

This work has been published as an article in the journal Cellular and Molecular Bioengineering.

Kheradmandi, M., Ackers, I., Burdick, M.M., Malgor, R. & Farnoud, A.M. Targeting Dysfunctional Vascular Endothelial Cells Using Immunoliposomes Under Flow Conditions. *Cellular and Molecular Bioengineering*, **13**, 189-199 (2020).

Introduction

Cardiovascular disease is currently the leading cause of death in the United States, with more than 840,000 new cases annually.[61] Atherosclerosis refers to the process of plaque formation within the walls of the arteries and is a multifactorial disease involving both genetic and environmental causes. Atherosclerosis plaques form by lipid accumulation in the intimal region of an artery, under dysfunctional endothelium monolayers.[81] This endothelial injury causes the accumulation of both monocytes and T-cells to the affected endothelium.[82] Following adhesion, monocytes migrate into the subendothelial space and transform into cholesterol-laden cells. The inflammatory responses are amplified by the increased number of local macrophages, commonly known as foam cells, which further contribute to the progression of the atherosclerosis plaque, thereby aggravating the disease.[83]

Despite the high incidence and clinical importance of atherosclerosis, the current treatment options for the disease are insufficient. Current standard drugs induce undesirable effects such as insulin resistance and type II diabetes.[84] Also, the plasma elimination half-life of atorvastatin, fluvastatin and other statins are shorter than 16 hours, due to protein-binding in the serum and rapid take-up by the liver.[85,86] This has led to increasing interest in the development of targeted strategies for treating atherosclerosis. Yoon et al.[87] have conducted an *in vitro* fibrin targeting study under static condition. In this experimental study, cysteine-arginine-glutamic acid-lysine-alanine (CREKA) conjugated nanoparticles have displayed almost 8 times increased targeting efficiency compared to the control micelles.[87] In another study, Winter et al.[88] focused on utilizing solid nanoparticles for specific delivery of drugs to the site of atherosclerotic plaques. However, the use of solid nanoparticles, such as paramagnetic perfluorocarbon leads to slow release of drugs as the particles degrade to release intracellular content.[88] While other nanocarriers have been examined for drug delivery in atherosclerosis, such studies have generally used non-biodegradable carriers,[34] focused on targeting macrophages, which are underneath the endothelium and not directly accessible to nanoparticles,[89] or examined *in vitro* cultures in static conditions,[90,91] not considering the fact that atherosclerotic plaques are subject to blood flow.

It is known that the endothelial cell surface of atheroma overexpresses vascular cell adhesion molecule 1 (VCAM1).[35,36,92] This molecule has already been utilized in a few drug delivery efforts. Sun and colleagues have studied conjugation of an atherogenic miRNA inhibitory drug to the surface of anti-VCAM1 functionalized gold nanospheres for delivery to endothelial cells.[37] Our group has also previously shown the possibility of targeting VCAM1 for delivery of solid particles to the site of atherosclerotic plaques.[34] Soft particles have also been investigated for VCAM1 targeting. The *in vitro* and *in vivo* specificity of anti-VCAM1 functionalized peptide amphiphiles have been studied by

Mlinar et al.[38] In addition, Pan et al.[39] have investigated the *in vivo* targeting of anti-VCAM1 functionalized perfluorocarbon nanoparticles in the mouse models of atherosclerosis. Given the promise of soft particles for drug delivery by targeting VCAM1, it is possible that a liposomal system could be advantageous in the context of drug delivery in atherosclerosis, given that drug release in liposomes upon their cellular uptake is faster than solid particles.[43] However, prior to utilizing liposomal nanocarriers for drug delivery in animal models of atherosclerosis, it is important to ensure that such carriers are not toxic to cells associated with the plaque, are capable of targeting dysfunctional endothelium, and that targeting can be achieved under both static and dynamic conditions.

In the current study, a liposomal formulation, conjugated to antibody against VCAM1, was evaluated for its ability to target inflamed human umbilical vein endothelial cells (HUVECs), under both static and dynamic conditions. The liposomal system was not toxic for macrophage or endothelial cells in–vitro and was able to target both fixed and non-fixed endothelial cells overexpressing VCAM1 in static conditions. Endothelial cell targeting was observed at almost the same level for medium with and without erythrocytes under flow (4 dyn/cm^2), albeit to a lower degree compared to static conditions. These results suggest that liposomal systems could be potentially used for drug delivery in animal models of atherosclerosis, which is a focus of future studies.

Experimental Section

Materials

Dioleoyl-phosphatidylcholine (DOPC), sphingomyelin (SM), cholesterol (Chol), and phosphatidylethanolamine-polyethylene glycol (2000 kDa)-cyanur (DSPE-PEG(2000)-Cyanur) were purchased from Avanti Polar Lipids (Alabaster, AL, USA). Sephadex G-25 in PD-10 desalting columns were purchased from GE Healthcare (Buckinghamshire, UK). Human Umbilical Vein Endothelial (HUVEC) Cells (C2519A) and EGM-2 BulletKits media (CC-3162) were purchased from Lonza (Allendale, NJ, USA). Human erythrocytes (SER-PRBC) were purchased from ZenBio (Research Triangle Park, NC, USA). Mouse normal IgG and polyclonal anti-vascular cell adhesion molecule1 (anti-VCAM1) antibody were purchased from Abcam (Cambridge, MA, USA). Goat anti-mouse IgG, mouse IgG1 kappa isotype control and FITC conjugated VCAM1 antibody and trypan blue stain were purchased from Thermo Fisher Scientific (Waltham, MA, USA). Chloroform, phosphate-buffered saline (PBS), Tris buffer and other solvents were purchased from Sigma (St. Louis, MO, USA).

Liposome Preparation

Liposomes were synthesized by hydrating dry lipid films. Lipid solutions were made by dissolving DOPC, SM, Chol, and DSPE-PEG (2000)-Cyanur (31.67:31.67:31.67:5 mol%) in chloroform. Liposomes were synthesized using the established freeze-thaw method, as shown in **Figure 1**.[93]

Figure 1

Schematic of Liposome Preparation using the Freeze-Thawing Technique.

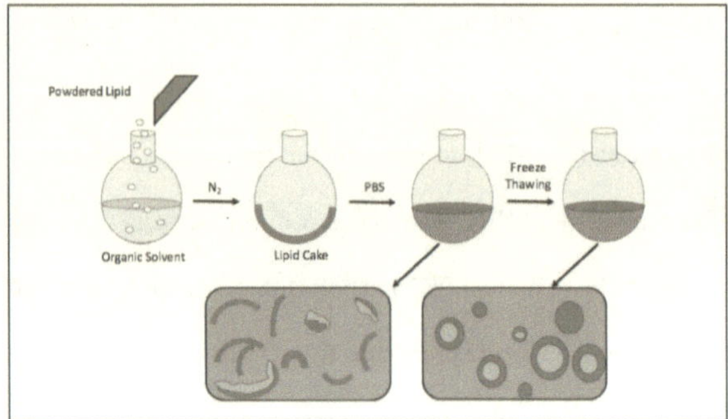

Briefly, lipid mixture was dehydrated under nitrogen gas to obtain a thin lipid film on the wall of glass test tubes. Lipid film was rehydrated with PBS buffer followed by vortex mixing to obtain a liposomal suspension with a final concentration of 0.2 mg/ml. The process was completed using seven freezing and thawing cycles by freezing the lipid solution in a dry ice, acetone bath followed by thawing in water bath at 40 °C for 3 minutes. Characterization of size and surface charge of liposomes were measured using a particle sizer (Zeta Sizer Nano ZS, Malvern Instrument Inc., Worcestershire, UK).

Liposome Leakage Assay

The stability of liposome was studied by fluorometry using carboxyfluorescein (CF) as the fluorescent probe, as reported previously.[94] To encapsulate CF in the vesicles, lipid films were rehydrated using 80 mM CF solution dissolved in PBS. Encapsulation was completed after 7 cycles of freeze-thaw. Unconjugated CF was separated using the Sephadex PD-10 separation column. Stability of liposomes was investigated at 37 °C under stirring by monitoring the fluorescence intensity of the released CF at 517 nm, as shown in **Figure 2**.

Figure 2

Schematic of Liposome Stability Measurement Technique using the Fluorescence Self-Quenching Probe.

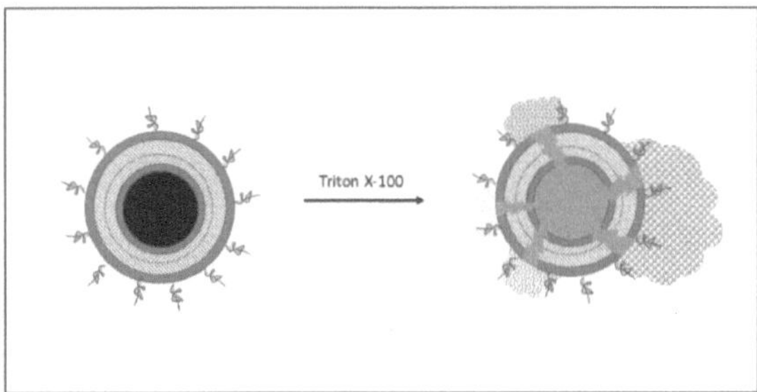

CF fluorescence is self-quenched when encapsulated inside liposomes at high concentration. Loss of liposome integrity over time results in the release of CF and an increase in fluorescence intensity. The total fluorescence intensity was obtained by disrupting the liposomes by adding 10 µl of Triton X-100 detergent in 2 ml of liposomal solution. The percentage of release at each sampling time was calculated by dividing the fluorescence intensity for that time point by the total release intensity of each experiment.

Liposome Cytotoxicity Study

Cytotoxicity of liposomes in HUVEC and THP-1 cell lines was evaluated using the Trypan Blue cell viability assay. In brief, confluent monolayers of HUVEC and THP-

1 cells were prepared in 6-well plates with specific media (EGM-2 and DMEM, respectively) and incubated with three different concentrations of liposome suspension (0.2, 0.02 and 0.002 mM). For the Trypan Blue assay, cells were exposed to liposomes for 12 or 24 hours. After incubation, cells were detached, using 0.025% trypsin solution, and collected. Trypan Blue staining was used to detect and count colorless viable cells with intact membrane, versus the distinctive blue dyed dead cells with damaged membranes.

Liposome Surface Functionalization

Antibody conjugation to the surface of liposomes was accomplished based on the direct-coupling method introduced by Bendas et al.[95] Direct-coupling process provides a stable covalent bond between the N-terminus of the antibody and the distal end of the PEG terminus on the surface of the liposomes. Briefly, liposomes were hydrated using the Tris buffer at a pH of 8.8 and normal mouse IgG was added at a 1:1000, antibody to lipid molar ratio, for 16 hours at room temperature. The unbound antibody was separated using centrifugation at 60000 g. Liposomes were washed twice using the Tris buffer.

A mouse IgG ELISA kit assay was used to determine antibody conjugation efficiency on liposome surfaces. This kit is an enzyme-linked immunosorbent assay for the quantitative measurement of mouse IgG conjugated liposomes using the horseradish peroxidase conjugated anti-mouse IgG detector antibody. Further characterization of antibody conjugation was performed using an confocal fluorescence microscope (ECLIPSE Ti, Nikon Instruments Inc.,Tokyo, Japan) with a 0.52 projection lens (Nikon Instruments Inc.,Tokyo, Japan) and 40x Fluor objective lens. To this aim, fluorescence microscopy was applied to analyze antibody liposome conjugation using the secondary fluorescent. DyLight-488 conjugated goat anti-mouse IgG was used at a 1:500 final volume dilution for 1 hour at room temperature. Rhodamine-DOPE (2 mol%) was incorporated in the liposome structure to allow for fluorescence visualization.

VCAM1 Expression Study

Previous studies have shown that lipopolysaccharide (LPS) can imitate inflammatory condition by inducing VCAM1 overexpression in endothelial cells.[33,96,91] A similar method was used in the current study to induce VCAM1 overexpression in HUVEC cells. HUVEC cells were seeded on 10 mm glass coverslips and cultured for 24 hours in a 6 well plate. Cells were treated with 100 ng/ml of LPS in the culture medium for 24 hours. Afterwards, cells were fixed with formaldehyde and incubated with FITC conjugated anti-VCAM1 at a 1:200 final volume dilution for 30 minutes in PBS. Then, cells were imaged using a Nikon A1R confocal laser scanning microscope system and the expression of VCAM1 was estimated by measuring the level of the fluorescence (FITC) intensity, using the ImageJ software.[97] Cells not treated with LPS were used as negative control. Kappa fluorescent antibody was used as an isotype antibody for positive control.

Liposome Targeting under Static Conditions

In order to stimulate VCAM1 surface overexpression, HUVEC cells (passage number 3–8) were cultured in a 35-mm tissue culture plate and treated with LPS (100 ng/ml) for 24 hours prior to the experiment. The specificity of the anti-VCAM1 functionalized liposomes to LPS-stimulated HUVEC cells was analyzed by measuring the final liposomal localization. HUVEC cells were seeded on glass cover slips and treated with 100 ng/ml LPS for 24 hours. Cells were fixed with paraformaldehyde and incubated for 30 minutes with 0.2 mM liposome suspension in PBS solution under static culture conditions at room temperature. Liposomes included 2 mol% rhodamine-DOPE in their structure to allow for fluorescence visualization. Studies were repeated without fixation to ensure that cell fixation, and the resulting protein crosslinking by formaldehyde, did not artificially modify binding. For these studies, cells were incubated with functionalized liposomes (0.2 mM) for 6 hours at 37°C before fixation to compare liposome targeting between fixed and non-fixed cells by confocal macroscopy with the rhodamine-based fluorescent measurement using the ImageJ software.

Liposome Targeting under Flow Condition

A three-dimensional, well-controlled flow chamber device was used to study liposome targeting to endothelial cells under flow conditions. Also, the possible interaction of functionalized liposomes with human red blood cells was investigated by adding erythrocytes, at 40% hematocrit (i.e. erythrocyte volume/total volume) into the flow chamber. A silicon rubber gasket was used to produce a cut-out channel with 0.5 cm width and 178 μm depth with a polycarbonate cover on top of gasket, using a previously established method.[98] This transparent polycarbonate disk was placed on top of the cell culture dish and provided a leak-proof seal using a vacuum pump to allow fluorescent microscopic visualization. **Figure 3** shows a schematic of this targeting experiment.

Figure 3

Schematic summary of the liposomal targeting mechanism under flow condition.

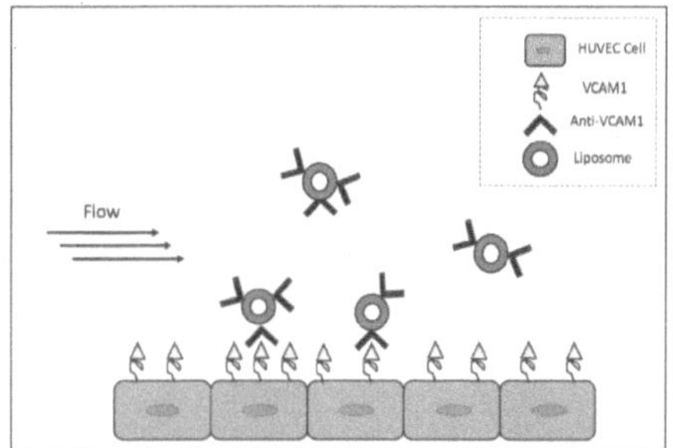

Fluorescent (rhodamine-conjugated) liposomes were suspended in EGM medium (0.2 mM) and perfused over HUVEC cells for 3 minutes with an average shear stress of 4 dyn/cm^2, as a representative shear stress for arterial blood flow in atherosclerosis lesion-prone.[99] An inverted-stage microscope (Leica, DMI6000B) with ×0.55 projection lens (Leica Microsystems, Mannheim, Germany) and 10x fluor objective were used to study liposomes targetability at room temperature and 4 dyn/cm^2 wall shear stress in the described system. Finally, fluorescence microscopy images were analyzed with ImageJ to quantify localized liposomes after washing the cells with pure medium flow for 30 seconds.

Results

Size and Charge Characterization of Liposomes

Liposomes were composed of three lipid components: dioleoyl-phosphatidylcholine (DOPC), sphingomyelin (SM), and cholesterol (Chol). This lipid composition was selected because of their biocompatibility, biodegradability and low toxicity.[100,101] They were characterized for size and charge at 37°C using dynamic light scattering. Liposomes had a mean diameter of 201.3 ± 3.3 nm and a surface charge of -7.7 ± 2.6 mV, and a narrow size distribution as determined by size distribution graphs, in PBS at 7.4 pH (**Figure 4**).

Figure 4

Characterization of liposome size distribution, showing the overlay of three independent size distribution measurements by dynamic light scattering in PBS, pH of 7.4 at 37 °C. The experiment was repeated six times.

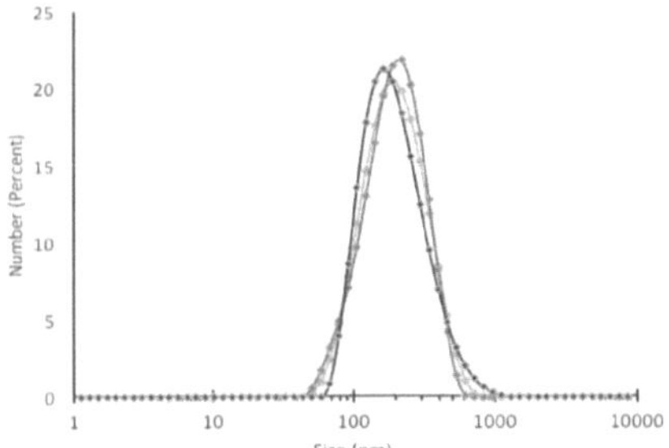

This liposome composition was selected due to its stability at physiological temperature, as shown in **Figure 5**. PEG groups were incorporated in the liposomal structure, as PEGylation is known to increase the circulation time *in vivo*.[26]

Stability Study of Liposomes

Liposomes were characterized for their stability at 37°C using laser Doppler anemometry. The stability of liposomes at 37 °C was examined by monitoring the release of the self-quenching fluorescent dye, CF, from their lumen. This study showed that almost 7% of CF was released from the liposomes after two hours of incubation in PBS (**Figure 5**), suggesting minimal release of the liposome content prior to uptake by cells, which has been reported to take more than 15 minutes following intravenous injection.[34]

Figure 5

Characterization of liposome stability as measured by the release of the self-quenching probe, CF, from the lumen of the vesicles in PBS, at 37° C, and pH of 7.4. Error bars represent the standard deviation of six measurements.

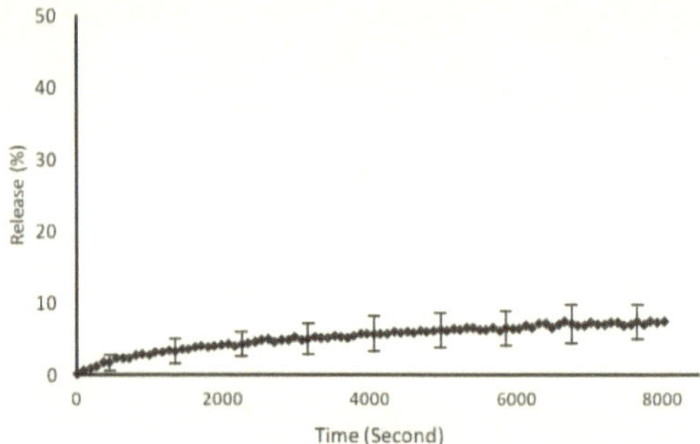

Cytotoxicity Study of Liposomes in THP-1 and HUVEC Cells

Next, the effect of liposomes on cell viability was examined in two of the major cell types found in atherosclerotic plaques, macrophages (derived from THP-1 monocytes), and endothelial cells (HUVEC). The Trypan Blue exclusion assay, which examines membrane integrity, was used to evaluate cell viability after exposure to liposomes. Cells were exposed to liposomes at various concentrations (0.002, 0.02, 0.2 mM) and cell viability was examined for 24 hours using the Trypan Blue dye. Also, the cellular metabolic activity of THP-1 cells was investigated using the MTS assay for up to 5 days after incubating them with liposomes. This assay confirmed the lack of cytotoxicity by liposomes (**Figure 6A, 6B and 6C**). The cell viability, for both THP-1 and HUVEC cells, remained at approximately 100% for 24 hours after the exposure to all concentrations of liposomes (**Figures 6A** and **6B**).

Figure 6

*Cell cytotoxicity of liposomes for **(A)** HUVEC and **(B)** THP-1 cells as measured by the Trypan Blue assay; and **(C)** cell cytotoxicity of liposomes for THP-1 cells as measured by the MTS assay. Bar graphs show liposome viability for not-treated cells and cells treated with 0.002, 0.02, and 0.2 mM of liposomes. The experiment was repeated six times and error bars represent the standard deviation of three independent experiments.*

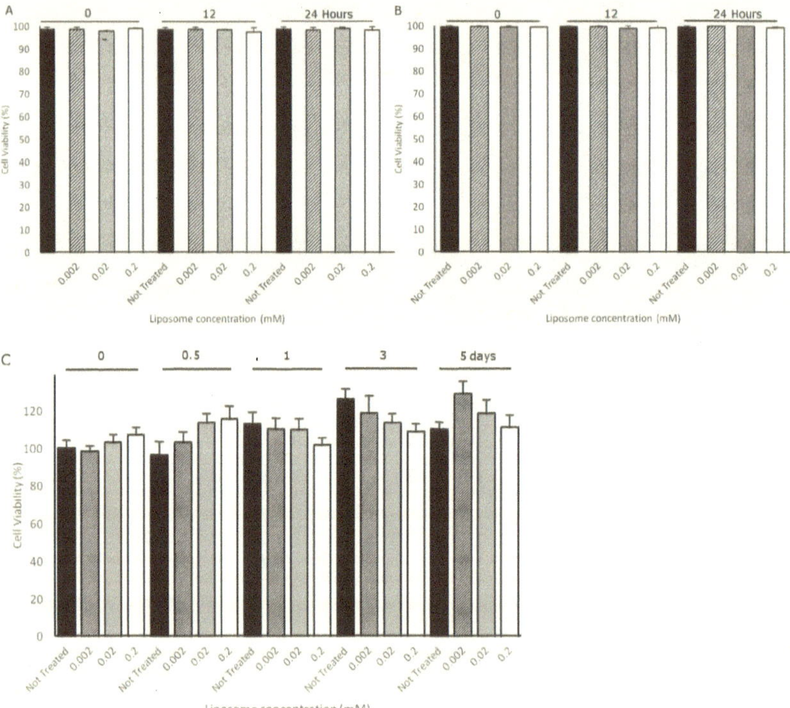

Surface Conjugation Efficiency of Liposome Functionalization

Upregulation of VCAM1 in the endothelial cell has been shown to be directly related to the process of the plaque formation and the pathogenesis of atherosclerosis.[102] Therefore, this cell surface motif could be a suitable target for site-specific delivery. To prepare a VCAM1-specific delivery system, liposomes were functionalized by coupling anti-VCAM1 antibody to the PEG terminus of liposomal surface in a molar ratio of 1:1:1:0.16 (DOPC:SM:Chol:DSPE-PEG-Cyanur). Quantification of antibody–liposome coupling efficiency was performed using the mouse IgG antibody. Antibody conjugation to cyanur in DSPE-PEG-cyanur was achieved by incubating the liposomes with the antibody at a protein:lipid ratio of 1:1000 for 16 hours at room temperature.[103] Excess, unconjugated antibodies were separated via centrifugation and removed after two Tris solution washes. Conjugation was confirmed using an ELISA assay kit to measure antibody conjugation to liposomes. A conjugation efficiency of 57.8 ± 8.4% was determined from the absorption spectrum of samples at 450 nm and total initial antibody concentration. This coupling efficiency is similar to the previously published coupling range which has been reported to be between 30% to 50% antibody-liposome binding efficiency.[95,104,105]

Conjugation of antibody to the surface of the liposomes was also examined using confocal microscopy. For this experiment, a FITC-conjugated secondary antibody was added to functionalized liposomes. Microscopy images showed significant co-localization between rhodamine (red) and fluorescein (green), which respectively represent labeled liposomes and FITC-conjugated secondary antibody (**Figure 7- left**

column). This co-localization of liposomes and secondary antibodies further confirmed antibody conjugation to the surface of the liposomes. In addition, liposomes showed significant uptake in THP-1 macrophages (**Figure 7- top right column**). No secondary antibody localization was observed in THP-1 cells when secondary antibodies were added to cells without conjugating them to functionalized liposomes (**Figure 7- middle column**).

Figure 7

Conjugation of normal mouse IgG antibody (AB1) to the surface of liposomes as examined by confocal fluorescence microscopy on a background of THP-1 cells. Cells were stained with DAPI (blue), while liposomes were stained with rhodamine (red), and the secondary antibody (AB2) was conjugated to FITC (Green). The top row shows successful conjugation of antibody to the surface of the liposomes, as well as the uptake of liposomes in THP-1 macrophages. Bottom row shows liposomes not conjugated with normal mouse IgG antibody, in which no binding of the secondary antibody was observed. Samples *were imaged at 60X magnification and scale bar=25 µm. The experiment was repeated six times.*

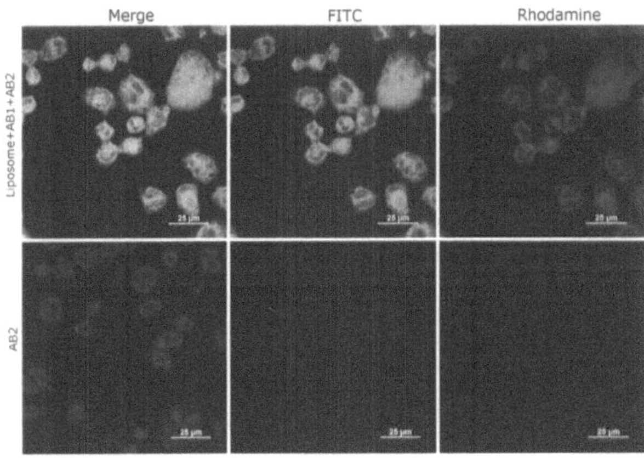

Expression Study of VCAM1 in Normal and Inflamed HUVEC Cells

VCAM1 overexpression in HUVEC cells was stimulated using LPS treatment to mimic pro-inflammatory conditions in atherosclerosis,[91] which results in VCAM1 upregulation. Incubating HUVEC cells with 100 ng/ml LPS for 24 hours led to significant VCAM1 expression. This was confirmed by incubating HUVEC cells with anti-VCAM1 antibody, followed by a FITC-conjugated secondary antibody, and measuring the FITC fluorescence signal (**Figure 8A**). This fluorescence signal was quantified based on the percentage of fluorescent pixels in these images, divided by the total number of counted cells. VCAM1 expression level of LPS-activated HUVEC cells was approximately 12 times more than un-treated cells and significantly higher than all other groups (**Figure 8B**). FITC-conjugated isotype control (Kappa antibody) samples illustrated significantly lower fluorescence pixels, demonstrating negligible non-specific binding.

Figure 8

(A) *VCAM1 expression in LPS-treated (100 ng/ml), left column, or untreated, right column, HUVEC cells. Confocal imaging with FITC (green) staining for anti-VCAM1 secondary antibody and Kappa isotype antibody.* Samples *were imaged at 40X magnification and scale bar=25 μm.* ***(B)*** *Fluorescence intensity measurement using the ImageJ software based on the number of green pixels per number of cells, indicating relative expression of cellular VCAM1. NC-LPS0: Negative control cells without LPS treatment, NC-LPS100: Negative control cells with 100 ng/ml LPS treatment, Iso-LPS0: Isotype Kappa secondary antibody without LPS treatment, Iso-LPS100: Isotype Kappa secondary antibody with 100 ng/ml LPS treatment, VCAM1-LPS0: VCAM1 secondary antibody without LPS treatment, VCAM1-LPS100: VCAM1 secondary antibody with 100 ng/ml LPS treatment. The experiment was repeated six times and error bars represent the standard error and **** indicates p<0.00001.*

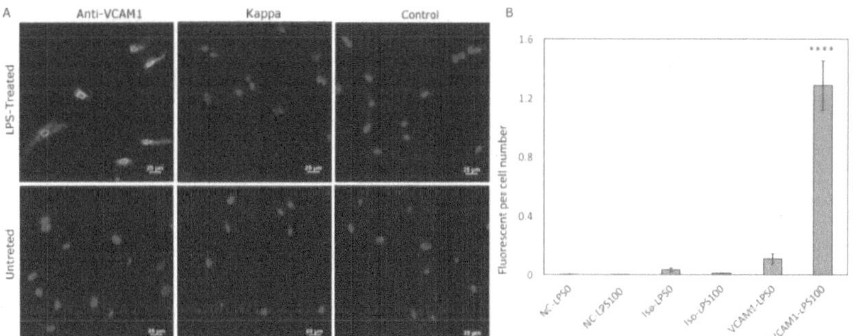

Functionalized Liposomes for Targeting Study under Static Condition

Anti-VCAM1 conjugated liposomes were used to target LPS-treated HUVEC cells overexpressing VCAM1. To this aim, LPS-treated and non-treated endothelial cell monolayers were prepared, fixed, and incubated with unfunctionalized (negative control), mouse IgG-functionalized (isotype control), and VCAM1-functionalized liposomes for six hours at 37 °C. The fluorescent lipid, rhodamine-DOPE, was incorporated in the structure of all liposomes to allow for fluorescence observations. Liposome localization with LPS-treated or non-treated cells was evaluated using confocal microscopy and quantified by dividing the percentage of pixels showing rhodamine fluorescence by the total cell number, labeled with DAPI, using the ImageJ software. VCAM1-functionalized liposomes showed at least 20 times higher localization to HUVEC cells compared to non-functionalized liposomes or liposomes functionalized with isotype control (**Figures 9A** and **9B**). Liposome co-localization was only observed when HUVEC cells were treated with LPS, demonstrating that localization was due to the overexpression of VCAM1, leading to successful targeting of liposomes to the LPS-treated HUVEC cells. Importantly, targeting was not limited to fixed cells. When the experiment was repeated for HUVEC cells that had not been fixed, an even higher extent of localization, ~67% higher compared to fixed cells, between VCAM1 functionalized liposomes and LPS-treated cells was observed (**Figures 9A** and **9B**).

Figure 9

Functionalized liposome localization in normal (non-treated) and LPS-treated (100 ng/ml) HUVEC cells. ***(A)*** *Confocal imaging showing liposome attachment to, or internalization in, HUVEC cells for anti-VCAM1-conjugated liposomes, isotype (IgG)-conjugated-liposomes, and liposome with no antibody attachment (negative control or NC). Cells were stained with DAPI (Blue) while liposomes were stained with rhodamine (Red).* Samples *were imaged at 40X magnification and scale cale bar=25 μm.* ***(B)*** *Quantification of results in A for both fixed and not-fixed HUVEC cells based on the fluorescence intensity measurements using the ImageJ software. Lip-LPS0: Cells treated with control unfunctionalized liposomes, without LPS treatment; Lip-LPS100: Cells treated with control unfunctionalized liposomes, and 100 ng/ml LPS treatment; Iso-LPS0: Cells treated with isotype antibody functionalized liposomes, without LPS treatment; Iso-LPS100: Cells treated with isotype antibody functionalized liposomes, and 100 ng/ml LPS treatment; and VCAM1-LPS0: Cells treated with anti-VCAM1-functionalized liposomes, without LPS treatment; VCAM1-LPS100: Cells treated with anti-VCAM1-functionalized liposomes, and 100 ng/ml LPS treatment. The experiment* *was repeated six times and error bars represent the standard deviation of the measurements. * and ** indicates $p < 0.05$ and $p < 0.01$, respectively.*

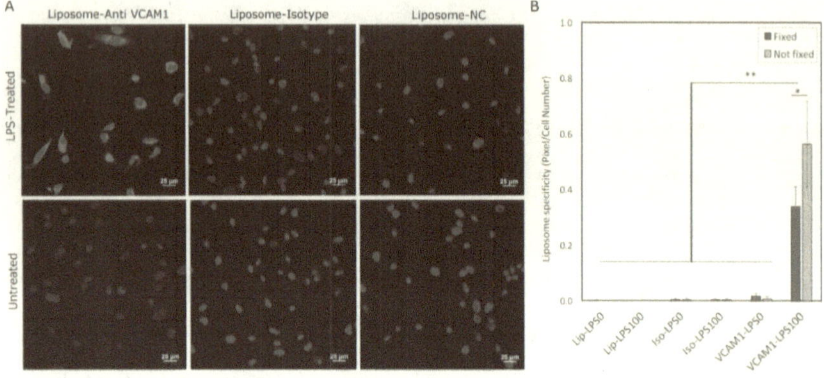

Functionalized Liposomes for Targeting Study under Flow Condition

Studies with VCAM1-functionalized liposomes confirmed successful targeting of HUVEC cells overexpressing VCAM1 in both fixed and non-fixed conditions. To examine targeting under shear flow, a parallel plate flow chamber, as described in the study of Shirure et al.,[98] was used. High expression of VCAM1 in HUVEC cells was again stimulated using LPS treatment (100 ng/ml) after HUVEC cells were cultured for 24 hours in 35 mm cell culture dishes. Then, the specificity of functionalized liposomes to VCAM1 was analyzed by suspending rhodamine-labeled liposomes, in the EGM medium used to grow HUVEC cells, and perfusing them using a syringe pump for 3 minutes over HUVEC cells. A shear stress of 4 dyn/cm^2, representative of the arterial vessel regions with higher risk of forming carotid atherosclerosis plaque was used,[99] followed by 30 seconds of washing with the cell culture medium. Liposome targeting was determined by confocal imaging and evaluating the fluorescence of bound liposomes using the ImageJ software. These results showed significantly higher localization of anti VCAM1 functionalized liposomes in LPS treated cells, compared to untreated cells, isotype control, and unfunctionalized liposomes. However, functionalized liposomes showed about 6-fold lower localization under flow condition compared to the static culture. This finding confirmed the high targeting capacity of VCAM1-functionalized liposomes to the surface of the inflamed HUVEC cells under both static and simulated blood flow condition. To evaluate whether blood components might affect the binding of liposomes to the site of the plaque, experiments were performed under shear flow in the presence of erythrocytes. No significant difference in the binding of vesicles to LPS-treated epithelial was observed in the presence or absence of erythrocytes (**Figure 10B**), indicating that the presence of erythrocytes does not disturb the ability of vesicles to target VCAM1.

Figure 10

Localization of functionalized liposomes under flow condition in normal (non-treated) and LPS-treated (100 ng/ml) HUVEC cells in the presence of erythrocytes (Medium + erythrocytes) or in their absence (Medium). ***(A)*** *Confocal imaging and staining with Rhodamine (Red) for liposomes for anti-VCAM1-conjugated-liposomes, isotype (IgG)-conjugated-liposomes and non-functionalized liposomes (control).* Samples *were imaged at 40X magnification and scale bar is 100 μm.* ***(B)*** *Fixed and not-fixed HUVEC cells targetability study based on the fluorescence intensity measurement using the ImageJ software for Lip-LPS0: Cells treated with control unfunctionalized liposomes, without LPS treatment; Lip-LPS100: Cells treated with control unfunctionalized liposomes, and 100 ng/ml LPS treatment; Iso-LPS0: Cells treated with isotype antibody functionalized liposomes, without LPS treatment; Iso-LPS100: Cells treated with isotype antibody functionalized liposomes, and 100 ng/ml LPS treatment; and VCAM1-LPS0: Cells treated with VCAM1 functionalized liposomes, without LPS treatment; VCAM1-LPS100: Cells treated with VCAM1 functionalized liposomes, and 100 ng/ml LPS treatment. The* *experiment was repeated six times and error bars represent the standard deviation of the measurements and *** indicates $p < 0.001$.*

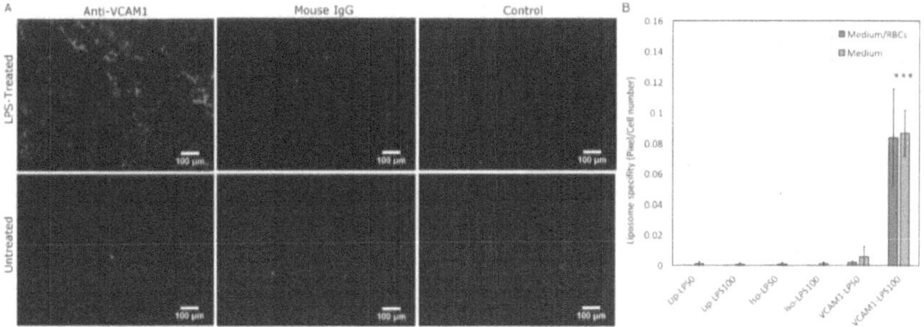

Discussion

In this study, development and characterization of a liposomal system for targeting of inflamed endothelial cells has been reported. The developed liposomes do not cause toxicity toward endothelial and macrophage cells and are able to maintain sufficient stability for targeting under blood flow condition. These liposomes, functionalized with antibody against VCAM1, were able to successfully target HUVEC cells overexpressing this protein under both static and dynamic conditions.

In developing liposomes for targeting atherosclerotic plaques, two important factors need to be considered. First, it is important for liposomes to not "leak" their content prior to reaching the plaque, so as to avoid significant systemic side effect. This was examined by investigating the leakage of a fluorescent probe from the lumen of the vesicles, which was confirmed to be minor (7% release after 2 hours under stirring at 37°C in PBS, **Figure 5**). It should be noted that the intracellular release of the liposome content (i.e., after internalization) is expected to be significantly higher due to the cellular breakdown of liposomes.[21] Secondly, it is important to consider the role of macrophages. This is because of the presence of a significant number of macrophages and foam cells in atherosclerotic plaque, which play an important role in the early stage and progression of the aortic atherosclerosis. Therefore, liposomes targeting endothelial cells would likely interact with, or get engulfed by, macrophages covering these cells. The liposomal carriers developed in this study showed no toxicity to either macrophages (**Figure 6A**) or endothelial cells (**Figure 6B**), even though they were internalized by macrophages in significant numbers (**Figure 7**).

Previous studies have proven upregulation of endothelial VCAM1 from an early stage in atherosclerosis.[106,107] In the current study, overexpression of VCAM1 was induced by LPS treatment (**Figure 8**). LPS treatment is a common method to induce inflammation treatment,[108] and has been used in a few previous studies to examine the role of VCAM1 and other adhesion molecules in myocardial dysfunction.[109,35,110,111] While LPS treatment did not cause any observable toxicity in HUVEC cells in the current study, potential unwanted adverse effects on cellular function due to LPS treatment cannot be ruled out. Anti VCAM1-conjugated liposomes showed significant localization inside and on the surface of HUVEC cells (**Figure 9**). Importantly, this binding was higher in non-fixed samples compared to fixed samples. This is expected as formaldehyde fixation is known to alter receptor-ligand interactions;[112] however, this finding is important as it implies that potentially higher targeting could be achieved *in vivo* where cell surface receptors are not structurally modified by the presence of fixatives.

While many studies have focused on cellular targeting by liposomes *in vitro*, the effect of shear flow on the efficiency of targeting is generally overlooked. In the current study, addition of shear stress in a parallel plate flow chamber decreased liposome localization in HUVEC cells by approximately five-fold. This effect could be attributed to the shear flow resulting in breaking the antibody-ligand binding or lower accessibility of the ligands in flow conditions. Previous studies have reported that shear stress affects and disrupts the function of the receptor-ligand bonds on the cell membrane.[109,113,114] Flow conditions have been shown to induce differences in the expression of adhesion molecules,[115] which can explain the difference in liposome localization. However, contrasting results also exist. Evans et al. have suggested that the introduction of flow increase the catch-bond characteristics of VCAM1 bonds on the plasma membrane.[116] While it is possible that shear stress enhances the catch-bond property of VCAM1 receptors, the results of the current study show a significant reduction in liposome binding and internalization under flow conditions. It is possible that the increase in the catch-bond is not significant enough to hold the liposomes after perfusion has been applied. This is in line with the study of Finger et al.,[117] demonstrating that T lymphocytes form stable tethers in a VCAM1 functionalized surface in a flow chamber, in shear stress values lower than 1.8 dyn/cm^2, but increasing the shear stress reduces bond stability. Therefore, VCAM1 bonds are sensitive to fluid shear stress *in vitro* and may vanish at higher shear stress values.

Due to the abundance of erythrocytes in blood, it is important to consider and explore their possible interactions with nanoparticles designed for therapeutic delivery. Simulation approaches have demonstrated that the tumbling movement of erythrocytes in blood vessels increases nanoparticle dispersion in the vein, thereby increasing nanoparticle concentration closer to the vessel wall.[118] The level of nanoparticle binding to the walls increases by ~50% after the addition of erythrocytes to the system. Therefore, we investigated the effect of erythrocytes on the ability of functionalized liposomes to target endothelial cells overexpressing VCAM1 was examined. However, the presence of erythrocytes did not affect the ability of functionalized liposomes to bind to HUVEC cells overexpressing VCAM1, with no statistical difference observed in the experiments with or without erythrocytes (**Figure 10**).

Taken together, our results indicate anti-VCAM1 antibody-functionalized liposomal system can effectively target inflamed endothelial cells overexpressing VCAM1 adhesion molecules under static and physiologically relevant conditions. Future studies are needed to examine the potential therapeutic application of this endothelium-targeting delivery system by encapsulating drugs to target and reverse or delay the progression of atherosclerosis.

Chapter 3: Cell-Derived Plasma Membrane Vesicles as a Drug Delivery System

Introduction

Functionalized liposomes used in our previous study have shown great ability to localize target cells (Chapter 2).[119] Liposomes, in general, became helpful in various experimental and biological applications due to their unique physical properties that resemble biological membranes.[100] Nonetheless, in comparison to the complexity of the cell membrane, the arrangement of lipids and proteins are comparatively simplistic in the manufactured system, and the information gained from this model system is restricted.[16] Additionally, liposomes are composed of only lipids and lack membrane proteins. Membrane proteins are one of the very critical features of cells to control the membrane thickness, transport nutrients, and control the exogenous interactions.[120] While protein incorporation seems like a possible solution; it is impossible for all practical purposes.

On the other hand, there is a severe lack of knowledge about the exact composition, position, order, and compartmentalization of proteins in the cellular plasma membrane.[121] Besides, the plasma membrane is constantly rearranging, shifting, moving, and changing bilayer composition in response to environmental and internal circumstances. All told, it is difficult to mimic this narrow (5 to 10 nm), unstable and complicated cellular compartment.[122] Therefore, plasma membrane synthesis from scratch is not a practical technique to obtain an ideal biomimetic delivery model.

Cell membranes are an advanced source of materials for molecular delivery systems. Cell membrane-derived vesicles, much more so than synthetic lipid or polymeric nanoparticles, have a multicomponent characteristic that includes lipids, proteins, and carbohydrates.[123] Due to their high functionalities and signaling platform similarities to the intact cell membrane, they can address various in vivo challenges, including the ability to minimize the immune system reaction.[124] The hollow-core structure of cell membrane-derived vesicles makes them a suitable coating material for different hydrophilic and hydrophobic pharmaceutical nanostructures. Cell membrane-derived vesicles have been used to coat a variety of therapeutic nanoparticles made of various materials and sizes, in addition to embedding small molecules within their exteriors.[125]

Drugs encapsulated in cell membranes have been shown to have a long-term, sustained release pattern. For the past three decades, red blood cells have been researched as delivery mechanisms for the ability to load and release various therapeutics, such as nucleic acids or synthetic drugs.[126,127,128] Mishra et al. have monitored the release of doxorubicin from red blood cell vesicles; the release study showed more than half of encapsulated drug was released slowly in the first 16 hours of incubation.[129] Although several small molecules, such as doxorubicin,[129] azidothymidine, and ethambutol,[130] have been encapsulated in the core of erythrocytes, larger drug macromolecules and nanoparticles have proven challenging to encapsulate due to lower uptake and higher membrane disruption.

Cell membrane isolation and reconstruction is also another technique that has gained much attention during the last decade.[131],[132] However, isolation of plasma membrane from other cellular organelles is a complex and time-consuming process which is requires the use of high pressures, sonication, strong chemicals, and/or detergents.[133] Unsurprisingly, the disruption of functional membrane components, especially the folding of membrane proteins, has been reported during very long detergent or sonication-based membrane isolation techniques.[134] Therefore, a new isolation technique would be greatly beneficial to obtain valuable information regarding the nanoparticle-plasma cell membrane interaction without the interference of the endocytotic process.

Giant plasma membrane vesicles (GPMVs) are micron-sized vesicles with the closest approximation to the size (<6 μm) and composition of the native plasma membrane. GPMVs hold promises for various applications, including research on coexisting fluid phases and membrane properties, which were previously performed on liposomes.[16] Due to the high similarity with biological membranes, they are also a promising candidate for drug encapsulation and delivery by limiting the potential toxicity and containing all membrane proteins, which could facilitate cellular uptake, targeting, and intracellular trafficking of cargos.

Trams et al. were first identified cell membrane-derived, extracellular vesicles as delivery and intercellular communication tool in 1981.[135] Some researchers have already shown few small molecules, and amphiphilic quantum dots can penetrate using the translocation process of peptides across the membrane into the lumen of GPMVs without the assistance of endocytic processes.[57],[57],[136] In one of these studies, Saalik et al. demonstrated that GPMVs could encapsulate small cell membrane penetrable peptides by direct translocation across the plasma membrane.[56] Another study with Pae et al.

confirms the previous finding while suggesting that proteins contribute significantly to the uptake of these small cell-penetrable peptides.[57]

However, these studies indicated that uncharged, negatively charged, or low positive charged peptides and dextran did not penetrate into the vesicle lumen.[56] Also, several phase segregation was reported after the direct membrane penetration method; the authors concluded that the peptide transportation could rearrange and change the lipid ordering of membranes. More importantly, the larger peptides with the molecular mass of 2–3 kDa or higher, or low drug concentration solutions did not show any considerable transduction using the direct membrane penetration process.[56,57] Considering all of this, a new loading mechanism is required to provide the encapsulation mechanism for bigger or not highly positively charged entities.

This study herein introduces a novel loading mechanism using parental cell uptake before vesiculation. The cell-derived GPMV system used in this study was generated by chemically inducing vesiculation in A549 alveolar epithelial cells. By feeding fluorescent, negatively charged, large nanoparticles (50 nm) to cells prior to GPMV generation, I have been able to generate a novel GPMV-based, core-shell, nanoparticle-vesicle structure. This system was evaluated for its size and charge, stability, lipid and protein composition, uptake, and toxicity in two types of mammalian cells, A549 and THP1 cells.

Experimental Section

Materials

Promega CellTiter 96™ Aqueous One Solution Cell Proliferation Assay (MTS), HEPES buffer, KCl, $CaCl_2$, and NaCl were purchased from Fisher Scientific (Pittsburgh, PA). Rhodamine-DOPE was purchased from Avanti Polar Lipids (Alabaster, AL). Sephadex G-25 in PD-10 desalting columns were purchased from GE Healthcare (Buckinghamshire, UK). Fluorescein isothiocyanate-conjugated plain, carboxyl-, and amine-modified silica nanoparticles (50 nm) were purchased from Micromod Partikeltechnologie GMBH (Rostock, Germany). Dithiothreitol, chloroform, methanol, phosphate-buffered saline (PBS), paraformaldehyde, and other solvents were purchased from Sigma (St. Louis, MO). A549 alveolar lung carcinoma cells were purchased from the American Type Culture Collection (Manassas, VA). Antifade mounting media with DAPI was purchased from the Vector Laboratories (Burlingame, CA).

Preparation and Characterization of GPMVs

RPMI 1640 supplemented with 10 volume% fetal bovine serum (FBS) was used for A549 cell culture. GPMVs were generated as described previously by Levental et al.[15] In brief, confluent monolayers of adherent A549 cells in a 100 mm tissue culture dish were washed three times with PBS buffer and stained with 0.1 mg/ml rhodamine-DOPE for 10 minutes at room temperature. Then, cells were washed three times using the GPMV buffer containing 10 mM HEPES, 150 mM NaCl, and 2 mM CaCl2. After washing, cells were incubated with 27.6 mM paraformaldehyde and 1.9 mM dithiothreitol vesiculation agents at 37 °C for one hour under gentle stirring. Then,

GPMVs were separated from the rich cellular supernatant with centrifugation at 500 rcf for 5 minutes. Also, two PBS washes following the centrifugation at 20,000 rcf for one hour at 4 °C were performed to separated GPMVs as a pellet at the bottom of the centrifuge tube. Then blebs were imaged to investigate their size using the confocal microscopy method.

Nanoparticle Encapsulation in GPMVs

To evaluate the ability of GPMVs to encapsulate intracellular content, I have added nanoparticles to the parent cells prior to the generation of GPMVs. Briefly, cells were first cultured at a 100 mm culture dish to reach a confluency of approximately 70% and pre-incubated with 0.05 g/l FITC conjugated carboxyl-modified silica nanoparticles (50 nm) for six hours, resulting in nanoparticle internalization, washed three times with PBS, and then chemically induced for GPMV generation in 27.6 mM paraformaldehyde and 1.9 mM dithiothreitol at 37 °C for one hour. GPMVs were separated as described above, with two PBS wash and two centrifugations. Confocal fluorescent imaging was used to confirm the encapsulation of nanoparticles inside the GPMVs.

GPMV Membrane Integrity Study

The membrane integrity of GPMVs was evaluated using the stability assay of entrapped fluorescent nanoparticles. The stability of GPMVs at 37 °C was examined by monitoring the release of the fluorescent nanoparticles from their lumen. Encapsulation of silica nanomaterials inside the A549 cell membrane-derived GPMVs was performed as described in the previous section. GPMVs were separated by centrifugation of GPMV-rich supernatant at 500 rcf for 5 minutes, washed three times with PBS, and harvested at

20,000 rcf for one hour and resuspended in the mounting media. Droplets of the nanoparticle-loaded GPMV solution were placed on a glass slide, incubated at 37 °C, and imaged using confocal microscopy after 1, 3, 12, 24, and 48 hours of incubation time.

Quantitative Analysis of the GPMV Lipidome and Proteome Profile

I then investigated alterations in the proteomic and lipidomic profiles of GPMVs after the encapsulation of silica nanoparticles. A549 cells were cultured in 100 mm culture dishes to 70% confluency and chemically induced for vesiculation. Nanoparticle-loaded and unloaded GPMVs were harvested at 500 rcf for 5 minutes and washed three times at 20,000 rcf for one hour and dried under vacuum for proteomic analysis at the Ohio State University Proteomics Facility (Columbus, OH).

Lipidomic samples were also prepared with an extra lipid separation step using the Bligh and Dyer method.[137] Briefly, nanoparticle-loaded and unloaded GPMVs were mixed with 2.5:2.5:1.25:1 molar ratio of CHCl3:MeOH:water:sample followed by vortexing and centrifugation at 1000 RCF for 10 minutes. The organic phase was separated and dried under nitrogen gas for the mass spectrometry-based lipidomic investigation at the Kansas State University (Manhattan, KS).

Membrane-Based Carriers for Nanoparticle Delivery Systems

I then examined the uptake of GPMVs, loaded with carboxyl-modified silica nanoparticles, in A549 and THP-1-derived macrophage cells, using confocal imaging. THP-1 and A549 cells were both cultured in RPMI 1640 media with 10 volume% FBS. Then, THP-1 and A549 cells were stained using the 0.1 mg/ml rhodamine-DOPE for 10 minutes at room temperature. After the generation of nanoparticle-loaded GPMVs, 30 volume percent of the resulting vesicles from one 100 mm culture dish of parent cells were harvested as described before, resuspended in the cell culture media, and incubated in one well of 12 culture plates for 6 hours with THP-1 and A549 cells lines, washed three times with PBS, and placed on the glass slides with DAPI containing mounting medium for confocal fluorescent imaging.

Cytotoxicity Study of GPMV Vesicles

In the next step, I examined the effect of GPMVs, nanoparticles, and nanoparticle-loaded GPMVs on cell viability. Different nanoparticles were used, including the plain, carboxyl- and amine-modified silica nanoparticles. To this aim, A549 cells were grown to 70% confluency in a culture dish and incubated with nanoparticles, nanoparticle loaded-, and unloaded- GPMVs for 6, 24, and 48 hours. The nanoparticle binding and uptake efficiency were calculated 69.78 ± 21.08, as described below based on the average of three different nanoparticles; this yield was calculated based on the weight of the added nanoparticles compared to the samples after drying in the nanoparticle loaded-GPMVs.

Entrapment efficiency = $[(W_i - W_f) / W_i] \times 100$

where W_i is the initial nanoparticle weight and W_f is the nanoparticle weight after loading in GPMVs. According to this nanoparticle loading yield, I added 69.78 volume percent of 0.05 g/l nanoparticle solution and 10 volume percent of loaded- and unloaded-GPMVs extracted from 100 mm culture dishes into each well of 96 well plates. Then, the MTS in vitro cytotoxicity assay was used to measure cytotoxicity based on the colorimetric analysis of cellular metabolic activities at 490 nm. This cell-based toxicity experiment is a helpful tool to predict the potentially toxic effects of engineered membrane vesicles in cells.

Statistical Analysis

All experiments in this study had at least three individual replicates. One-way ANOVA with Dunnett's test was performed to compare different samples. Graphpad Prism software was used for statistical analysis (La Jolla, CA). For each experiment, the average and standard deviation were reported in the mean ± standard deviation format. P-values of 0.05 were considered statistically significant.

Results

Size and Charge Characterization of GPMVs

The chemical induction method was used to produce this cell-derived, core-shell system in A549 alveolar epithelial cells.[15] The resulting blebs were stained using the rhodamine-dope dye and imaged using Bradford and confocal microscopy techniques (**Figure 11A** and **11B**). Size measurement of GPMVs was performed using 10 confocal images. ImageJ software was used to measure the average diameter of 115 vesicles from 10 images. The average diameter was determined 5.7 ± 2.3 μm using ImageJ software. Also, dynamic light scattering method showed the average size of vesicles 4.9 + 1.4 μm. There is no statistically significant difference in the size measured using the ImageJ software and dynamic light scattering method. Since the surface charge has been shown to have a significant impact on the biodistribution of delivery systems,[138] I have used laser doppler anemometry to measure the surface charge of GPMVs. The surface charge of GPMVs was measured to be -29.4 ± 1.2 mV in PBS at 7.4 pH.

Figure 11

*Visualization of GPMVs derived from A549 cells using (**A**) Phase contrast microscopy and (**B**) Confocal microscopy imaging for Rhodamine (Red)-DOPE stained GPMVs.* Samples *were imaged at 100X magnification and scale bar is 5 μm. The experiment was repeated six times.*

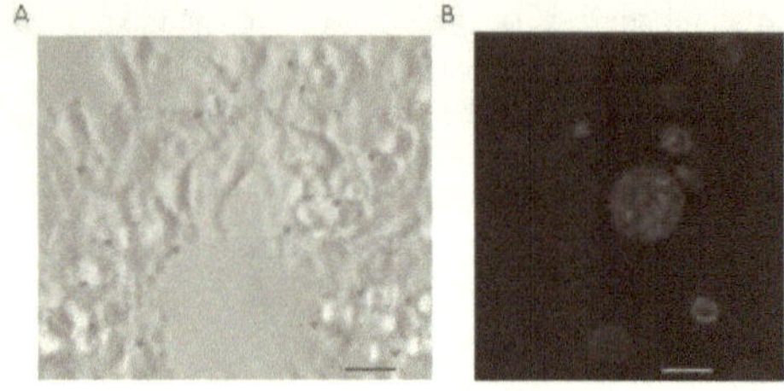

Encapsulation of Nanoparticles in GPMVs

Herein, a new loading mechanism was introduced by incubating nanoparticles with parental cells. This new loading mechanism relies on the capability of the parental cells to uptake nanoparticles by endocytosis and diffusion. Nanoparticles were first added to the culture media. Then, chemical induction was used to harvest the nanoparticle-loaded GPMV vesicles. Confocal imaging confirmed the presence of FITC-conjugated nanoparticles inside the Rhodamine-DOPE stained vesicles (**Figure 12**). This implies that silica nanoparticles were successfully uptaken by A549 cells using the active endocytic and passive diffusion and adhesive interaction pathways. Later during the vesiculation process, the cytosol content of parental cells, including the nanoparticles, was initially trapped into the vesicles before they shift to the cell membrane and excreted form the parental cells.

Figure 12

Internalization of nanoparticles in the A549 cells-derived GPMVs, examined by confocal fluorescence microscopy. GPMV membrane and silica nanoparticles were stained with rhodamine (red) and FITC (green), respectively. Samples *were imaged at 100X magnification and scale bar is 5 μm. The experiment was repeated six times.*

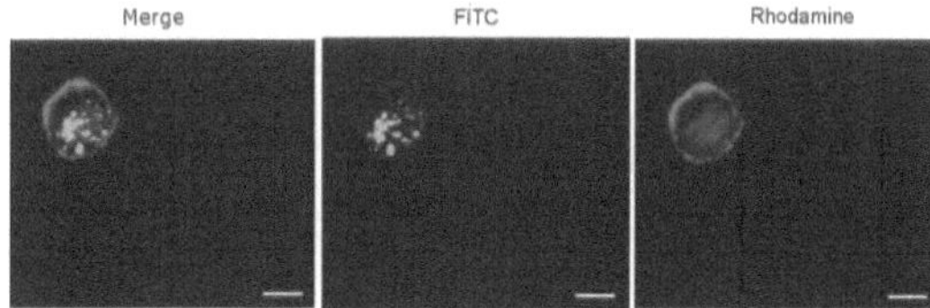

Stability Study of Nanoparticle-Encapsulated GPMVs

Pharmaceutical stability testing is a major criterion to separate the safe and reliable systems from undesirable fragile carriers. The thermal stability in the psychologically relevant condition and integrity duration were investigated for 48 hours in this study. To test the integrity of this cargo, FITC-conjugated GPMVs were vesiculated from A549 cells, as described before. Then, I incubated the slides containing loaded-GPMVs in the mounting medium at 37° C for up to 48 hours. Images clarified that nanoparticle encapsulated-GPMVs had spherical and intact shapes. This study proved that nanoparticles have remained encapsulated and stable inside the GPMV vesicles for at least 48 hours (**Figure 13**).

Figure 13

Stability study of nanoparticles encapsulated in GPMV after 48 hours as examined by confocal fluorescence microscopy. GPMV membrane and silica nanoparticles were stained with rhodamine (red) and FITC (green) stains, respectively. Samples *were imaged at 100X magnification and scale bar is 5 μm. The experiment was repeated six times.*

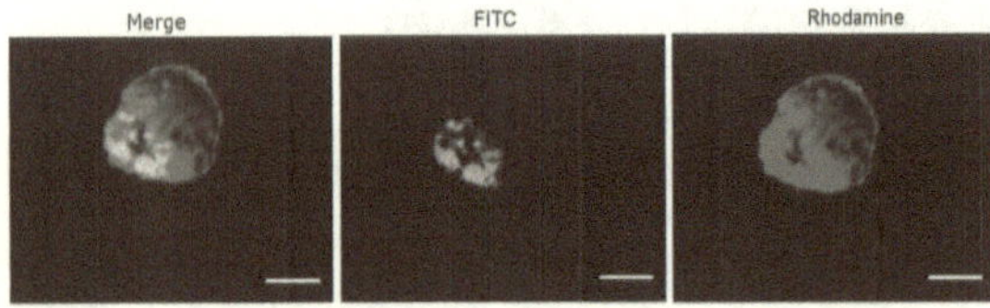

Lipidomic and Proteomic Analysis of GPMVs

A comprehensive understanding of the nanoparticle-GPMV interaction is necessary for the clinical translation of *in vitro* assessments. Lipidomic and proteomic techniques provide important insights into biochemical responses of cells by identifying and quantifying numerous lipids and proteins.[139] Lipid and protein profiling was applied here to investigate the potential impacts of encapsulating nanoparticles within the GPMV core-shell structure. A549 cells and carboxyl-modified nanoparticles were used to study the protein and lipid profiling of loaded- and unloaded-GPMVs. Vesicles showed the same lipid and protein profiles as reported for the cell plasma membrane with only minor changes in their lipidome and proteome, with or without encapsulation of nanoparticles. Lipidomics showed just one significant difference (decrease in ePC level) in the lipidome of nanoparticle-containing GPMVs (**Figure 14A**). Moreover, the protein abundance profile was consistent with the data reported by Eastlake et al. for normal retinae cells (**Figure 14B**).[140] Nanoparticle-membrane interaction caused two upregulated expressions in the glyceraldehyde-3-phosphate dehydrogenase (GAPDH) and human serum albumin (SPLAB) proteomes as compared to control unloaded GPMVs that may be caused by the intracellular nanoparticle corona. These results demonstrated that the lipid and protein composition of plasma membrane derived vesicles would not change drastically from exposure to silica nanomaterials.

Figure 14

Analysis of lipid- and protein- profile changes in silica nanoparticles loaded and unloaded GPMVs. (A) Comparative lipidomics analysis between the 13 most abundant lipids. (B) Proteomic profiling of all membrane proteins. The experiment was repeated *three times and error bars represent the standard deviation of three measurements. * indicates p < 0.01.*

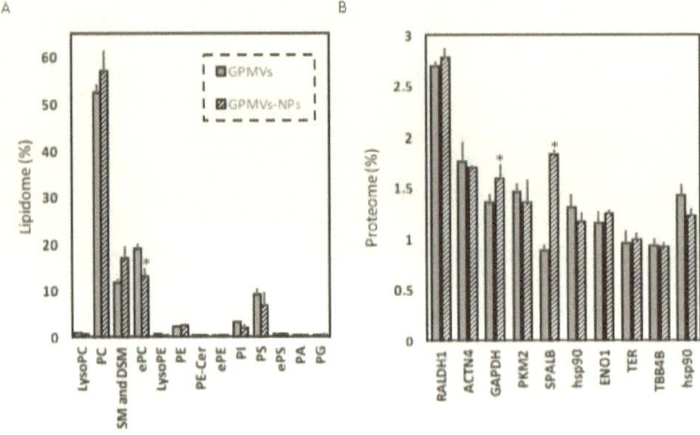

Cellular Uptake and Release of Nanoparticle Loaded-GPMVs

Cellular uptake of large macromolecules and drug carriers is generally ineffective. As a result, developing efficient delivery systems for intracellular delivery of chemical and biological substances is desirable. Confocal imaging indicated that nanoparticle encapsulated GPMVs were readily endocytosed in A549 (**Figure 15-top rows**) and THP1 cell lines (**Figure 15-bottom rows**). Higher recipient cellular uptake level was observed for encapsulated nanoparticles compared to the other control groups, including the nanoparticles, GPMV (not shown here), and control cell groups. Therefore, GPMVs can effectively facilitate delivering cargo to multiple cell types and can potentially serve as a novel drug/nanoparticle delivery system.

Figure 15

GPMV internalization in A549 and THP1 cells as examined by confocal fluorescence microscopy. The plasma membrane and nucleus of adherent A549 cells were stained with rhodamine (red) and DAPI (blue), respectively, while silica nanoparticles were stained with FITC (Green). Four different groups were imaged for each cell type, including the nanoparticle, GPMV (not shown here), *nanoparticle encapsulated GPMV, and control cells.* Samples *were imaged at 60X magnification, and scale bar is 25 μm. The experiment was repeated three times, and NP denotes silica nanoparticles.*

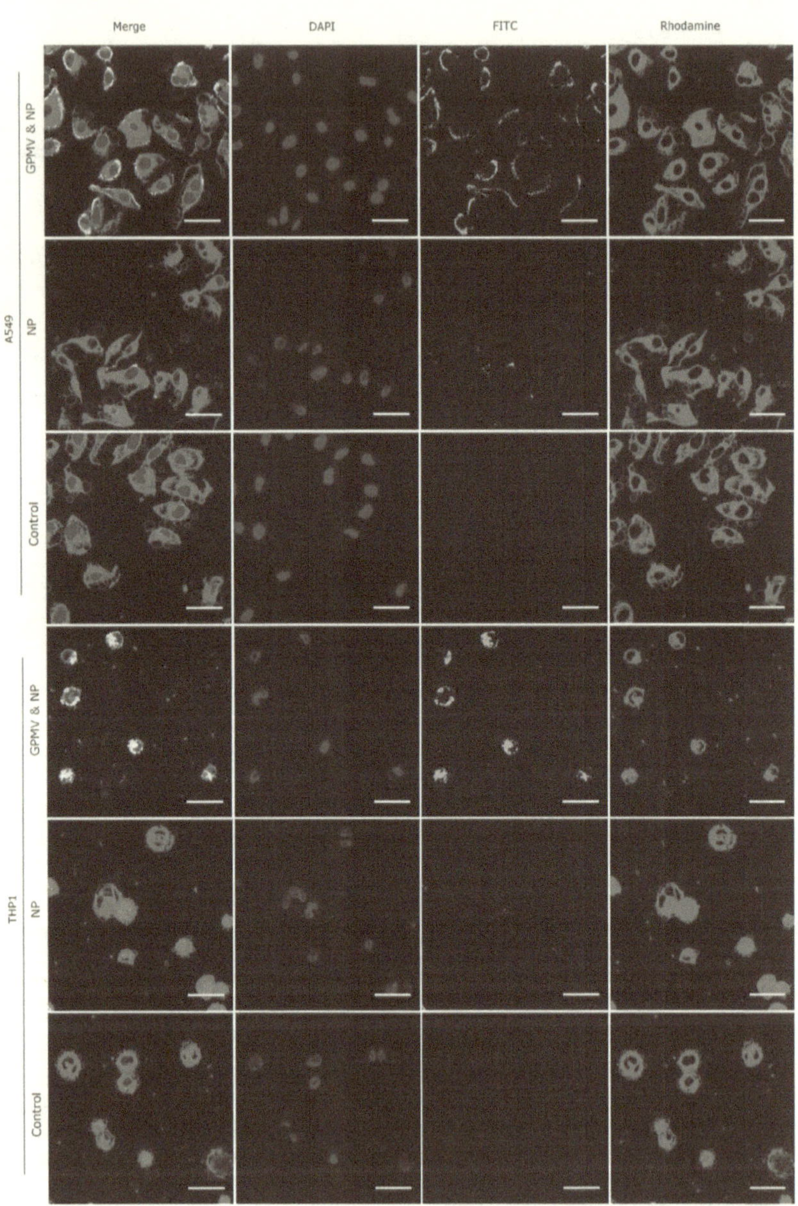
Merge
DAPI
FITC
Rhodamine
A549
GPMV & NP
NP
Control
THP1
GPMV & NP
NP
Control

Cytotoxicity Study of Nanoparticle Loaded and Unloaded GPMV Vesicles

The size and charge of plain, carboxyl-, and amine-modified silica nanoparticles (50 nm) were measured using the dynamic light scattering and laser Doppler anemometry at 0.05 g/l in PBS at 7.4 pH (**Table 1**). The nominal size of purchased nanoparticles was compatible with the size measured using the dynamic light scattering technique.

Table 1

The hydrodynamic diameter and zeta potential of different surface-modified nanoparticles in PBS at 7.4 pH. The experiment was repeated three times.

Sample	Size (nm)	Charge (mV)
Plain Nanoparticle	49.6 ± 10.1	-19.4 ± 3.8
Amine Coated Nanoparticle	50.1 ± 10.5	-18.5 ± 1.4
Carboxyl Coated Nanoparticle	52.1 ± 8.4	-16.7 ± 1.6

The cytotoxicity of silica nanoparticles encapsulated in cell membrane-derived carriers was first compared to control cell membrane vesicles alone and free nanoparticles. Measured via the MTS assay, the control GPMV vesicles did not cause any toxicity, similar to the untreated control cell. Free carboxyl modified silica nanoparticles did not show any significant toxicity either. Plain nanoparticles showed significant toxicity starting from 6 hours ($p < 0.01$). Amine-modified silica nanoparticles began to show significant toxicity after 24 hours ($p < 0.1$). Adding cell membrane-derived shells decreased the cellular toxicity in all groups, especially for plain nanoparticles (**Figure 16**). These findings confirm that GPMV vesicles are able to deliver toxic nanoparticles with reduced cytotoxicity compared to free nanoparticles, even at concentrations that would otherwise be significantly toxic.

Figure 16

*Effect of GPMVs and different nanoparticle-loaded GPMVs on A549 cell viability as examined by MTS assay for 6, 24, and 48 hours. Plain, amine and carboxyl modified nanoparticles was used to measure cytotoxicity based on cellular metabolic activities measured by the MTS assay. The experiment was repeated three times and error bars represent the standard deviation of the measurements. *** indicates $p < 0.001$ and ** indicates $p < 0.01$..*

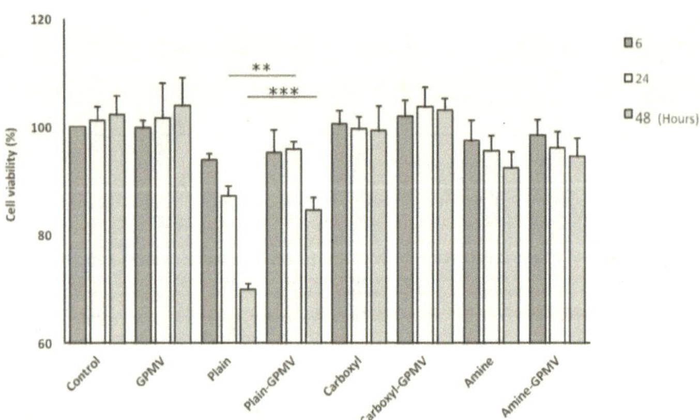

Discussion

Nanomedicine defines as the precisely engineered materials in the nanoscale to apply for novel therapeutic and diagnostic modalities.[141] Encapsulating nanomedicines within a biocompatible coating is a promising technique for resolving cytotoxicity, which is a major concern restricting the usage of several therapeutics.[142] Different natural, artificial and polymer-based delivery systems have been developed to provide safe passage, slow-release, and target delivery. While liposomes are the most widely used and well-studied nanocarriers for drug delivery,[143] cell membrane-based systems have been proved to offer better biocompatibility with little to no cytotoxicity than liposomes.[123]

A previously exciting finding indicated the possibility of loading highly positively charged peptides and cell penetrable compounds in a low loading efficiency within GPMVs.[57,56] However, this technique still excluded many potential therapeutic applications, including negatively charged nanoparticles.[56] Here, I have introduced a novel loading mechanism for large silica nanoparticles (50 nm). Carboxyl modified silica nanoparticles were used for the loading purpose with the zeta potential of -16.7, which is very close to the previously reported charge of -20.7 by Rocca et al.[144] In contrast to the previous claim with Saleek et al.,[56] I have successfully loaded these negatively charged nanoparticles in the core of cell membrane-derived shells (**Table 1**).

Parent cells, A549 cells, were incubated with negatively charged carboxyl modified nanoparticles. Then, GPMVs were vesiculated while entrapping the parental intracellular cytosol with 69.8 % nanoparticle loading efficiency (**Figure 12**). The nanoparticle entrapment yield is similar to the previously reported numbers.[145,146,147] In one of these studies, Belwal et al. have observed 71% loading efficiency for the encapsulation of silica nanoparticles inside the liposomes composed of phosphatidylcholine and polyethylene glycol (PEG-2000).[145] In another study, Lehi et al. have reported 71.4 % of silica nanoparticles (50 nm) inside the SBA-15 nanoparticles.[146]

Encouraged by the successful encapsulation result, I continued exploring this model to further characterize the membrane stability after encapsulating nanoparticles within them. The stability of drug delivery systems refers to the extent that a container can retain drugs and/or nanoparticles within specified space and throughout its period of storage and use.[148] Since leakage of delivery systems is an essential factor for the overall therapeutic index, I assessed the retention of nanoparticle encapsulated GPMVs over 48 hours at 37 °C. While some fluctuation of the membrane was observed, confocal images indicated nanoparticles remained trapped inside the cell membrane-derived vesicles (**Figure 13**). This result confirms the previously published leakage study by Saalik et al.,[56] which indicated that at least for one hour after cell membrane penetrable peptides were loaded inside the GPMVs, entrapped peptides did not release significantly into the media.

Lipidomics and proteomic techniques have provided several important biochemical insights into nanoparticles alternations of membrane-derived vesicles. They can be used as an early detection methods before most diseases or abnormalities get into the terminal stages.[149] Herein, I investigated any alteration in the lipid and protein profiling of cell membrane-based core-shell structure in response to the addition of nanoparticles. My study showed only a few alternations between hundreds of lipid and protein components (**Figure 14**). Therefore, the addition of carboxyl-coated silica nanoparticles to A549 cells did not cause considerable biochemical alternations in the cell membrane-derived vesicles.

Since several therapeutic paths are localized in subcellular compartments of recipient cells, it is critical to understand how drug carrier systems interact with desired cells and how the cargo-cell interaction affects cellular uptake and release.[150] Furthermore, drug carriers' uptake and final destination using different direct or via endocytosis entry is often the main parameter to determine the overall therapeutic efficacy, kinetics, and transferability to the animal model studies. Confocal imaging results indicated a strong uptake and uniform release of encapsulated nanoparticles inside the recipient A549 and THP-1 cells (**Figure 15**). This positive finding suggests the high biocompatibility of the proposed system in future *in vivo* applications.

In vitro cytotoxicity assays often measure the ratio of cellular death in direct response to nanoparticle addition, which is a critical part of new delivery systems development. Different nanomaterials exhibit different cytotoxicity within the same recipient cells based on their particular physical, compositional, cellular uptake, and membrane interaction.[151] Here, I have utilized three different plain, carboxyl-, and amine-modified silica nanoparticles to investigate the feasibility of using cell membrane-derived vesicles in reducing the cellular toxicity caused by these nanoparticles. MTS toxicity assay showed a different level of cell death in response to different nanoparticles. Also, GPMV vesicles have been proved to reduce the toxicity caused by nanoparticles significantly in plain silica nanoparticle-loaded GPMVs and enhanced A549 cell viability

(**Figure 16**). My observation regarding the plain silica toxicity is supporting the finding of several other published articles.[152,153,154] Diabate et al. have suggested that silica nanoparticles damage the integrity of plasma membrane and cellular metabolic activities.[153] Moreover, my results confirm the previously stated concept that surface modification using the amine and carboxyl groups has shown a significant improvement in the biocompatibility of silica nanoparticles.[154,155] I also noticed a significant reduction to no cytotoxicity after covering nanoparticles the cell membrane-derived vesicles.

In conclusion, my results and previous research show that various compounds, including large nanoparticles, can be loaded into GPMV vesicles to transported therapeutics into the recipient cells, implying that GPMVs may be used as great delivery systems with little to no cytotoxicity and high loading capacity due to their large macro sizes. Additionally, while GPMV vesicles lack the cortical cytoskeleton, endocytosis, and other biological processes powered, they still maintain the biochemical complexity of the native plasma membrane, including being composed of almost all the same lipids, proteins, and other matrix components, which distinguishes GPMV membrane models from other artificially made lipid vesicles and even live-cell membrane studies.

Chapter 4: Role of Membrane Proteins and Lipids in Nanoparticle Induced Cell Membrane Damage

Introduction

The cell plasma membrane acts as a biological filter to keep cellular constituents in; while allowing vital nutrients into the cell and holding undesirable contaminants and waste products out. The cell membrane defines the cell within the bilayer boundaries and decides the interaction with surrounding signals and entities. While the mechanisms of nanoparticle-induced toxicity are diverse, membrane damage is an established mechanism of toxicity by almost all solid particles.[156] However, it is widely recognized that much more progress is still needed in understanding the mechanisms of membrane toxicity, resulting from the exposure to solid particles. Lipid molecules account for about half of the mass of most mammalian cell membranes.[157] A 1 m x 1 m region of lipid bilayer contains approximately 5 x 10^6 lipid molecules in the plasma membrane.[158]

All membrane lipids are amphiphilic molecules with a hydrophilic polar head and a hydrophobic nonpolar tail. The amphipathic nature of membrane lipid molecules causes them to form liposomal bilayers spontaneously in aqueous environments.[158] The fluidity of different lipid bilayers is influenced by the composition as well as the location and arrangement of its different subregions.[158] The hydrophilic head is composed of choline and a phosphate group connected to glycerol with two hydrophobic tails called fatty acids. Fatty acids differ in length between 14 and 24 carbon atoms.[159] Usually, one of the tails is unsaturated with one or more cis-double bonds, which form a small kink in the unsaturated tail.[160] The capacity of phospholipid molecules to pack next to each other is essential for the order and fluidity of the membrane, which is deeply influenced by the variations in the number of carbon atoms and saturation of the phospholipid tails.[161]

Several in vitro experiments have been conducted to determine the impact of fatty acid saturation on the biophysical properties of the synthesized membrane models (liposomes). These previous studies indicated that unsaturated fatty acids' length and structural properties could restrict lipid ordering within model membranes.[161,162,163] Although liposomes are commonly used as a membrane model to examine nanoparticle-induced membrane toxicity, the observations in liposomes do not always translate to mammalian cells due to the fact that liposomes cannot mimic membrane lipid diversity and the presence of membrane proteins.

Altogether, the plasma membrane offers a basis of association for different membrane lipids and proteins.[120] The membrane component proportions vary with cell type, but generally, nearly all of the remaining 50 percent of most human cell components by mass is composited of proteins.[164] Proteins are large, water-soluble, highly charged molecules directly associated with the overall charge, polarity, lipid packing, and fluidity of plasma membranes.[165] While incorporating different proteins in the liposomal structures is a time-consuming and complicated process,[166] cell membrane-derived vesicles are a great biomimetic membrane candidate with all membrane proteins already embedded within their structure.

Here, I utilized GPMVs as a physiologically relevant model for the cellular plasma membrane. While GPMVs are not completely asymmetric, they mimic the diversity of membrane lipids and the presence of membrane proteins, allowing for a better understanding of the role of membrane proteins in nanoparticle-membrane interactions. Our results indicate that the addition of membrane proteins and saturation of membrane lipids contribute to the fluidity, charge, and integrity of the GPMV membrane, thereby affecting nanoparticle-membrane interactions.

Experimental Section

Materials

Fluorescent plain, amine, and carboxyl-modified silica nanoparticles with 50 nm nominal diameter were purchased from Micromod Partkeltechnologie (Rostock, Germany). Methyl-α-cyclodextrin was purchased from AraChem (Tilburg, Netherlands). Phosphatidylserines (POPS (16:0/18:1)) and 1,2-dipalmitoyl-sn-glycero-3-phosphoethanolamine-N-(7-nitro-2-1,3-benzoxadiazol-4-yl) (ammonium salt) (NBD PE (16:0)) were purchased from Avanti Polar Lipids (Alabaster, Al). 1-(4-trimethylammoniumphenyl)-6- phenyl-1,3,5-hexatriene p-toluenesulfonate (TMA-DPH), 1,6-Diphenyl-1,3,5-hexatriene (DPH), Roswell Park Memorial Institute (RPMI) medium 1640, 0.25% trypsin with EDTA, fetal bovine serum (FBS), and phosphate-buffered saline (PBS) were purchased from Thermo Fisher Scientific (Waltham, MA). A549 alveolar lung carcinoma cells were purchased from the American Type Culture Collection (Manassas, VA). Formaldehyde, DL-1,4-Dithiothreitol (DTT) were purchased from Fisher Scientific (Pittsburg, PA).

Preparation of Membrane Models

A549 cells were cultured, and GPMVs were produced from A549 cells as described before in chapter 3. Briefly, A549 cells at 70% confluency were washed three times with the GPMV buffer and incubated with 27.6 mM paraformaldehyde and 1.9 mM dithiothreitol vesiculation agents at 37 °C for one hour. GPMV vesicles were separated with centrifugation at 500 rcf for 5 minutes, three PBS washes, and final centrifugation at 20,000 rcf for one hour.

GPMV-like, protein-free vesicles were also synthesized to examine the role of membrane proteins in nanoparticle-induced membrane damage. To this aim, GPMVs were subjected to lipid extraction using the established Bligh and Dyer procedure.[137] Briefly, GPMVs were derived from A549 cells and mixed with methanol, water, and chloroform in the 2.5:2.5:1.25:1 molar ratio (CHCl3:MeOH:water:sample, respectively). This organic-water solution was vigorously vortexed for 10 minutes and centrifuged at 1000 RCF for 10 minutes. The bottom phase was separated and dried under the nitrogen gas. This procedure is expected to only isolate GPMV lipids without including any proteins. Extracted lipids were then formulated into vesicles by adding warm PBS solution at 40 °C to the lipid film, applying several vigorous vortexing steps, and completing seven cycles of freezing and thawing at 40 and -78 °C. Samples were suspended in the PBS solution at 7.4 pH. Protein-free vesicles were then extruded 10 times using 1 μm filter at 70 °C, and examined for the size and surface charge in the PBS solution using the dynamic light scattering and laser doppler anemometry.

Examining the Role of Proteins in Membrane Integrity

Plasma membrane proteins play key roles in regulating membrane integrity and permeability.[167] In this study, I have investigated the impact of proteins on the stability of plasma membrane by monitoring the release of cytosolic compounds overtime after exposing them to nanoparticles. Lactate dehydrogenase (LDH) kit is a widely used in vitro cytotoxicity assay for measuring the lactate dehydrogenase cytoplasmic enzyme using a lactate dehydrogenase enzyme biomarker.[168]

Here, I have studied membrane integrity in protein-containing GPMVs and protein-free, GPMV-like control vesicles with the same lipid composition but without proteins. The control vesicle (GPMV-like membrane) was formed directly from the extracted lipids of GPMVs. GPMV vesicles were prepared as described above; A549 cells were cultured in 100 mm dishes, washed three times with GPMV buffer, and vesiculated using the chemical induction at 37 °C for one hour.

GPMV membranes were pelleted by centrifugations at 500 rcf for 5 minutes, three washes with PBS, and another centrifugation at 20,000 rcf for one hour. Then, GPMV vesicles were exposed to plain, amine, and carboxyl modified nanoparticles at 0.05 g/L concentration in PBS solution for one hour. Every 10 minutes, 200 μl of GPMV solution that was almost equal to 2×10^6 vesicles per ml of solution was centrifuged at 20,000 rcf for one hour at 4 °C. Hemocytometer was used for estimating the vesicle count. Clear supernatants were then transferred into one well and incubated with 50 μl of LDH reaction mix for 30 minutes at room temperature. The disruption of each sample was measured at 450 nm. Pure PBS and 0.05 g/L nanoparticle solutions were centrifuged and incubated with LDH reaction mix and used as the background control.

Carboxyfluorescein (CF) loaded GPMV-like membranes were also made from the membrane lipids, which were extracted from GPMVs using the Bligh and Dyer method.[137] Protein-free vesicles were prepared using the extracted lipids and the freeze-thawing method, as described before.[119] The lipid film was rehydrated with 80 mM CF solution, extruded 10 times using the 1 μm filter at 70 °C, and separated using Sephadex PD-10 separation column from unconjugated CF. GPMVs and protein-free vesicles were dispersed in 0.05 g/L nanoparticle-PBS solution at the same membrane concentration (g/l) and incubated for one hour at 37 °C. Eventually, I investigated the potential disruption and release of internal cytosolic enzymes and CF probe for protein-containing and protein-free vesicles using the LDH assay and fluorometry techniques, respectively, every 10 minutes after 1 hour incubation time with nanoparticles at 37 °C.

Examining the Role of Proteins in Nanoparticle Binding to the Membrane

Studies have found that membrane adsorption regulates the cellular membrane toxicity level caused by nanoparticles.[169] Here, I investigated the role of membrane proteins in the adsorption of plain, amine, and carboxyl nanoparticles onto the membrane surfaces using flow cytometry and confocal fluorescence microscopy. Protein-containing model (GPMVs) was isolated from the A549 cells, and protein-free vesicle model was prepared using the extracted lipids from GPMVs. All membrane models were stained with rhodamine-DOPE for 10 minutes and washed three times with PBS buffer. Then, membranes were exposed to the fluorescent silica particles at 0.05 g/l concentration for one hour to investigate the membrane-nanoparticle disruption and interaction. Rhodamine-DOPE stained membranes were used as the control without exposing them to particles. Surface adsorption of nanoparticles was studied using the confocal fluorescence microscope and flow cytometry methods. Nikon Elements software was then used to quantify the nanoparticle-membrane colocalization and total membrane stained areas.

Exogenous Lipid Exchange Method

In recent years a surge of membrane studies has focused on understanding the function of the proteins and lipids in the membrane-nanoparticle interactions. To examine the role of lipids in membrane-nanoparticle interaction, I applied a recently introduced method by Li and colleagues to alter lipids in the outer leaflet of plasma membranes.[170] They have developed a novel lipid exchange method to manipulate the lipid composition of the living cellular membrane using methyl-α-cyclodextrin. Briefly, A549 cells at 70% confluency were washed three times with the GPMV buffer and incubated with 27.6 mM paraformaldehyde and 1.9 mM dithiothreitol vesiculation agents at 37 °C for one hour. GPMV membranes were separated with centrifugation at 500 rcf for 5 minutes, washed three times with PBS, and pelleted with another centrifugation at 20,000 rcf for one hour. Methyl-α-cyclodextrin was preincubated with 1.5 mM of the desired lipid, POPS, in RPMI at 70 °C. Then 40 mM lipid loaded methyl-α-cyclodextrin solution was incubated with GPMVs for one hour to exchange membrane lipids with POPS as the desired lipid. Eventually, methyl-α-cyclodextrin treated GPMVs were washed three times with PBS to remove the extra loaded methyl-α-cyclodextrin prior to resuspending the membrane vesicles for further studies.

Confirmation of Membrane Lipids Exchange

To confirm the lipid exchange, fluorescent lipid was exchanged on the vesicle membrane using the previously introduced technique with Vahedi et al.[171] Briefly; a 19:1 molar combination of POPS and 1,2-dipalmitoyl-sn-glycero-3-phosphoethanolamine-N-7-nitro-2-1,3-benzoxadiazol-4-yl (NBD-PE) was loaded into the methyl-α-cyclodextrin, and incubated with the GPMVs derived from A549 cells. This assay allows for identification, quantification, and comparison of lipid exchange in normal, POPS:NBD-PE loaded methyl-α-cyclodextrin treated, and only POPS:NBD-PE incubated vesicles using the confocal microscopy and Nikon Elements software techniques. A549 cells were cultured until 70% confluency and then vesiculated with chemical induction. GPMVs were separated and treated using the preloaded methyl-α-cyclodextrin. Intact GPMV membranes and GPMVs incubated with POPS:NBD-PE without methyl-α-cyclodextrin treatment were used as two controls in this assay.

Examining the Role of Lipids in Membrane Integrity

In this section, I examined the role of membrane lipids in nanoparticle–membrane interactions by varying membrane lipid composition. It has been already proven that the lipid composition of membrane models is a key characteristic in nanoparticle binding and membrane disruption.[172] Here, I applied an individual lipid exchange method to investigate the function of lipids in membrane integrity. A549 cells were cultured in 100 mm tissue culture dishes, washed three times with GPMV buffer, chemically vesiculated, and centrifuged for 5 minutes at 500 rcf, then washed three times with PBS, and centrifuged for one hour at 20,000 rcf.

Separated GPMVs were incubated with 40 mM POPS preloaded methyl-α-cyclodextrin for one hour. After three times of PBS washing, GPMVs were incubated with 0.05 g/L plain, amine, and carboxyl modified silica nanoparticle-PBS solution for one hour at 37 °C. The impact of POPS:NBD-PE exchange in the disruption of GPMV membranes was investigated using the confocal fluorescence microscope, LDH membrane integrity kit, and fluorometry techniques in the presence or absence of the POPS lipid exchange using the methyl-α-cyclodextrin treatment.

Examining the Role of Lipids in Nanoparticle Binding to the Membrane

Further investigation is necessary to determine the role of membrane lipids in regulating the interaction between nanoparticles and plasma membranes. Surface adsorption of nanoparticles onto the GPMV membranes after exchanging membrane lipids with POPS, revealed the role of POPS lipid in regulating nanoparticle-plasma membrane interactions. GPMVs were isolated from the A549 cells, as described before. Single lipid exchange was performed with 40 mM preloaded methyl-α-cyclodextrin for one hour at 37 °C. Intact GPMV membranes was used as the control group. GPMV membranes, with and without methyl-α-cyclodextrin treatment, was stained with rhodamine-DOPE for 10 minutes, and exposed to the fluorescent plain, amine, and carboxyl modeified silica nanoparticles at 0.05 g/L concentration for 1 hour. Then, adsorption of nanoparticles onto the membrane surfaces was studied using confocal fluorescence microscopy and flow cytometry methods. Quantification of surface adsorption was performed based on the expression area of nanoparticle-membrane colocalization and total membrane stained areas using the Nikon Elements Software.

Fluorescence Anisotropy

The degree of membrane disruption by nanoparticles has been shown to be related to cell plasma membrane fluidity.[173] As a result, more rigid membranes are expected to experience less damage. The role of membrane lipids and proteins in the fluidity of bilayer membrane was investigated by fluorescent anisotropy.

The fluorescence anisotropy value is a dimensionless number representing the ratio of the linearly polarized emission intensity to the whole emission intensity of the components. This ratio is inversely proportional to the fluidity of the cell membrane, as a high anisotropy value represents a low membrane fluidity. Anisotropy (r) is calculated using the fixed wavelength that excites to the rotatable excitation polarizer in both vertical and horizontal excitation positions using the equation below,

$$r = \frac{\frac{I_{VV} * I_{HH}}{I_{VH} * I_{HV}} - 1}{\frac{I_{VV} * I_{HH}}{I_{VH} * I_{HV}} + 2}$$

Where I_{VV} is the detected vertically polarized emission resulted by vertical excitation, and I_{VH} is the detected horizontally polarized emission resulted by vertical excitation. Then, the excitation polarizer will be rotated to calculate I_{HH} that is the detected horizontally polarized emission resulted by horizontal excitation, and I_{HV} that is the detected vertically polarized emission resulted by horizontal excitation.[174]

I expect to observe higher anisotropy, and lower disruption for membrane based on the selective incorporation of proteins. I also expect to get a higher fluorescence anisotropy value in the presence of higher saturated lipids in membrane composition which means a higher structural order.

Fluorescence Anisotropy of Both Bilayers

Measurements of membrane fluidity in both inner and outer leaflets were carried out using the fluorescent probe diphenylhexatriene (DPH) that is able to incorporate in the hydrophobic region in the bilayer.[175] To this aim, GPMVs were separated from A549 cells as described before. Protein-free vesicles were prepared using the extracted membrane lipids, GPMV-like vesicles, as described in the previous part. Also, lipid exchanged membranes were prepared using the methyl-α-cyclodextrin treatment, as described before. Then, 2 ml of DPH solution in acetone with 2 mM concentration was added and vortexed in 0.2 mol% to 2 ml of the intact protein-containing (GPMV), protein-free (liposome), and lipid exchanged vesicles in the PBS solution. The emission intensities were recorded by spectrophotometer at 430 nm for both samples, and the anisotropy was estimated using the difference in intensity of linearly polarized emission components to the initial intensity.

Fluorescence Anisotropy of Exterior Bilayers

Individual lipid exchange using the methyl-α-cyclodextrin treatment has been shown to only affect the outer leaflet of membranes.[171] Therefore, measuring the membrane fluidity in the outer leaflet can provide valuable information on how replacing the native lipid composition with the desired saturated lipid can affect the firmness of the membrane locally. TMA-DPH acts as a charged cationic analogue moiety that is unable of reaching the hydrocarbon areas after getting embedded inside the lipid bilayer. This molecule is tethered to the interface, while the DPH part of the molecule is oriented in the same line as other lipid within the bilayer.[176]

Figure 17

Schematics of TMA-DPH and DPH positioning, movement and orientation within the lipid membranes.

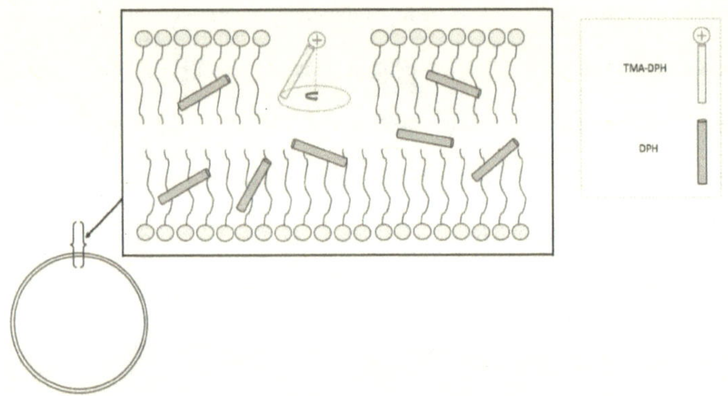

TMA-DPH was dissolved in methanol, added and vortexed in 2 ml of the intact protein-containing (GPMV), protein-free (liposome), and lipid exchanged vesicles in the PBS solution at a concentration of 40 nM. The emission intensity was recorded by spectrophotometer at 430 nm for both samples, and the difference in intensity of linearly polarized emission components to the initial intensity was used to calculate the anisotropy.

Statistical Analysis

At least three individual replicates were used in each experiment in this study. To compare different samples, a one-way ANOVA with Dunnett's test was used. For statistical analysis, the GraphPad Prism package was used (La Jolla, CA). The average and standard deviation for each experiment are reported in the mean standard deviation format. Statistical significance was defined as a P-value of 0.05.

Results

Characterization of GPMV and Protein-Free GPMV Membrane Models

Particle size and charge are two significant factors that play critical roles in the therapeutic index, especially the circulation and absorption.[177] The dynamic light scattering method was used to measure the size of protein-containing and -free GPMV vesicles. Size measurements showed the average size of vesicles 4.9 ± 1.4 µm for GPMVs and 1.3 ± 0.1 µm for protein-free GPMV membranes (**Table 2**). Variation in the particle surface charge affects the binding of vesicles to the cellular membrane, the uptake ratio inside the cell, and the final destination of nanoparticles in different cellular compartments both in vitro and in vivo.[177] Laser doppler anemometry was used here to measure the surface charge of protein-containing and -free GPMV Vesicles. Zeta potential analysis showed that the surface charge of GPMVs was less negative after removing the membrane proteins (**Table 2**). This observation confirms the previous study by Nishino et al. that indicated the ion exchange function and three-dimensional structure of proteins are important factors regulating the zeta potential of cell membranes [178]

Table 2

Hydrodynamic size and surface potential of GPMV and protein-free GPMV vesicles measured in PBS at 7.4 pH. The experiment was repeated three times to obtain the standard deviations.

Sample	Size (µm)	Charge (mV)
GPMV	4.9 ± 1.4	-29.4 ± 1.2
Protein-Free GPMV	1.3 ± 0.1	-13.0 ± 0.5

Examining the Role of Proteins in Membrane Integrity

Membrane proteins are responsible for the cell polarity and membrane structural stability by containing patches of hydrophobic amino acids where they interact with lipids in the membrane bilayer and patches of hydrophilic amino acids on surfaces that reach into the water-based cytoplasm.[165] Therefore, it is expected that vesicles containing proteins have better stability than protein-free vesicles. On the other hand, the chemically induced vesiculation technique is associated with multiple local ruptures during the blebbing process due to the high content of protein and cholesterol within their structure.[179] LDH kit was utilized to measure the loss of membrane integrity over time. Lactate dehydrogenase enzymes usually are compartmentalized within the plasma membrane wall, but the extracellular expression significantly increases in the extracellular medium in response to the loss of membrane integrity during cellular stress or death.

Here, intact GPMV vesicles showed more release after 1 hour of pre-incubation in PBS at 37° C due to the membrane ruptures (**Figure 18**). However, after the initial burst release, protein-containing vesicles were less leaky than protein-free vesicles, which can likely be explained by protein-lipid interaction. So, regardless of the primary burst release of internal contents, protein-containing GPMVs were 136% more stable after getting exposed to the plain silica nanoparticle (50 nm) than protein-free vesicles.

Figure 18

*Stability characterization of cell based vesicles for (**A**) protein-containing and (**B**) protein-free GPMVs as measured by the release of CF probe and lactate level from the lumen of the vesicles in PBS, at 37° C, and pH of 7.4. The experiment was repeated three times and error bars represent the standard deviation of at least three independent measurements.*

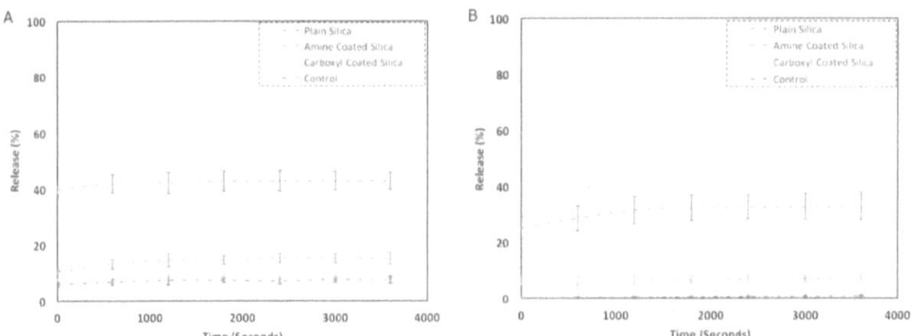

Examining the Role of Proteins in Nanoparticle Binding to the Membrane

The degree of membrane disruption is shown to be directly related to the nanoparticle adsorption on the membrane.[180] Since the zeta potential study showed a significant effect of membrane proteins in charge of the biological membrane (**Table 2**), it is essential to investigate the potential effect of proteins in nanoparticle-plasma membrane interaction. Confocal fluorescence microscopy was applied to visualize and quantify the colocalization of attached FITC-conjugated nanoparticles and rhodamine stained protein-containing and -free vesicles using the expression area measurement in the Nikon Elements Software. The difference in the surface adsorption of all three plain, amine, and carboxyl modified nanoparticles were significant between protein-containing and -free vesicles (**Figure 19B**). The quantification of surface adsorption study indicated that proteins significantly enhance nanoparticles and plasma membrane interaction. Additionally, confocal imaging showed that plain and amine-modified nanoparticles caused structural fluctuation and cracks in protein-containing GPMV vesicles, while the protein-free vesicles suffered unexpected changes in their morphologies.

Figure 19

Absorbance of plain, amine and carboxyl modified nanoparticles to the surface of protein-containing and -free GPMV vesicles derived of the A549 cells ***(A)*** *Confocal fluorescence microscopy of protein-containing GPMVs.* ***(B)*** *Quantified based on the area of colocalization of two fluorescent probes, green and red stain, per total red cell membrane area measurement using NIS Elements.* ***(C)*** *Confocal fluorescence microscopy of protein-free GPMVs.* Samples *were imaged at 100X magnification and scale bar is 5 µm in all images. Vesicles were stained with rhodamine (red), and nanoparticles were conjugated to FITC (Green). Control samples represent vesicles without nanoparticles. The experiment was repeated three times and error bars represent the standard deviation* *of the measurements. **, *** and **** indicates $p < 0.01$, $p < 0.001$ and $p < 0.0001$, respectively.*

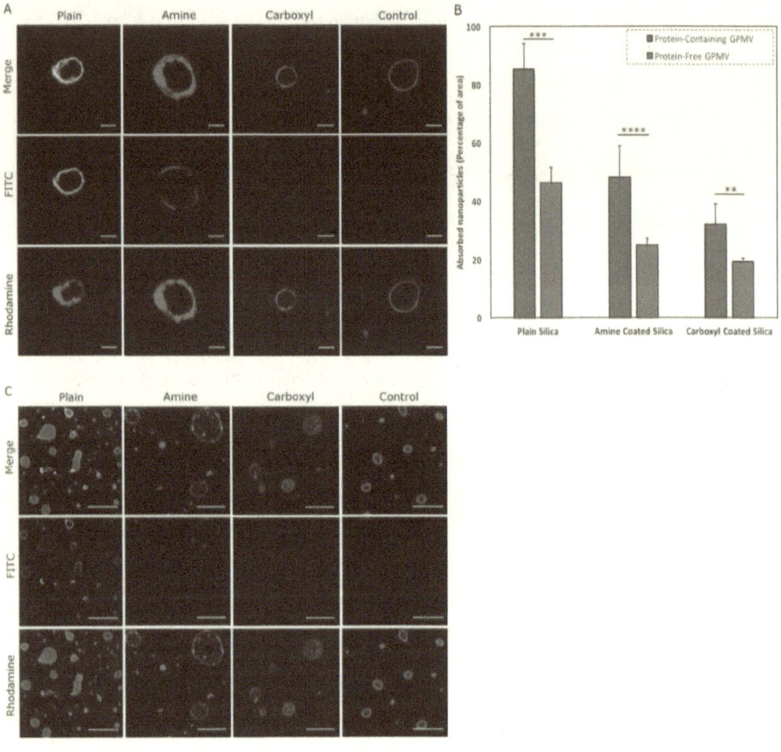

The membrane adsorption of nanoparticles was also investigated using the flow cytometry method. Protein-containing and -free models were isolated from A549 cells and stained using the rhodamine-DOPE fluorescent dye. Plain, amine-, and carboxyl-modified silica nanoparticles were monitored using their FITC conjugated stain. Flow cytometry results showed the same trend that was observed in the confocal microscopy technique (**Figure 20**). Both techniques indicate the importance of membrane protein in nanoparticle-cell membrane interaction. That is, the presence of proteins in the biological membrane increase the ability of biological membranes to interact and adsorb silica nanoparticles.

Figure 20

*Absorbance of plain, amine and carboxyl modified nanoparticles to the surface of protein-containing and -free GPMV vesicles derived of the A549 cells using the flow cytometry analysis. **(A)** Flow cytometry dot plots showing vesicle and nanoparticle populations for: **(1)** Dot plot analysis of protein-containing vesicles vs. plain nanoparticles. **(2)** Dot plot analysis of protein-containing vesicles vs. amine-modified nanoparticles. **(3)** Dot plot analysis of protein-containing vesicles vs. carboxyl-modified nanoparticles. **(4)** Dot plot analysis of protein-free vesicles vs. plain nanoparticles. **(5)** Dot plot analysis of protein-free vesicles vs. amine-modified nanoparticles. **(6)** Dot plot analysis of protein-free vesicles vs. carboxyl-modified nanoparticles. **(B)** Comparison analysis by flow cytometry for vesicle and nanoparticle positive population percentage (Q2 quadrant). The experiment was repeated three times and error bars represent the standard deviation of the measurements; * indicates p < 0.1.*

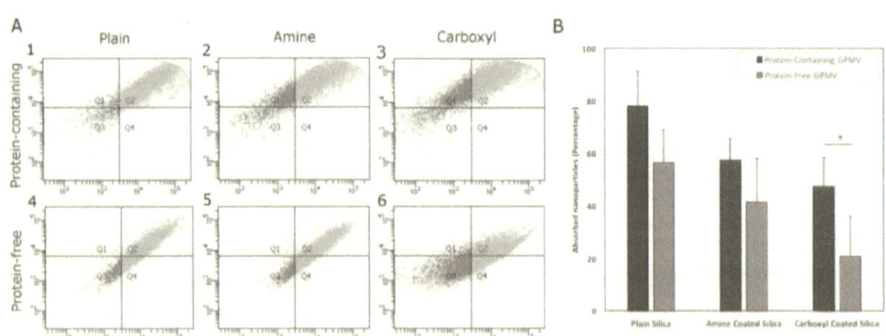

Exogenous Lipid Exchange Characterization

The single lipid exchange method was performed based on the previously introduced technique by Li et al.[170] The procedure involved pre-loading of methyl-α-cyclodextrin with the lipid of interest and replacing the exogenous lipids with the desired lipid, which takes place in the outer leaflet. Additionally, another study has shown that POPS loaded methyl-α-cyclodextrin did not cause considerable damage to the cellular membrane.[171] Altogether, I decided to exchange POPS with the exogenous membrane lipids to investigate the role of saturated lipid exchange in the physiochemical characteristics of biological membranes. The surface charge of vesicles was measured after lipid exchange using a laser doppler anemometry. Results showed that the exchange of membrane lipids with POPS decreased the surface charge of the vesicle (**Table 3**). This result confirmed the previously reported observation in the exchange of POPS lipid within human erythrocyte membranes.[181] Size measurements by dynamic light scattering did not indicate any significant size variation in the GPMV vesicles attributable to the exogenous lipid exchange.

Table 3

Hydrodynamic size and surface potential of GPMV and lipid exchanged GPMV vesicles measured in PBS at 7.4 pH. The experiment was repeated three times to obtain the standard deviations.

Sample	Size (μm)	Charge (mV)
GPMV	4.9 ± 1.4	-29.4 ± 1.2
Lipid Exchanged GPMV	4.9 ± 2.4	-33.3 ± 1.3

Confirmation of Native Membrane Lipids Removal after Lipid Exchange

Confocal microscopy was used to confirm that exogenous lipids were exchanged by methyl-α-cyclodextrin in the cell membrane outer leaflet. POPS and NBD-PE, the fluorescent lipid, were preloaded with methyl-α-cyclodextrin and incubated with vesicles in a 19:1 POPS:NBD-PE molar ratio. The same fluorescent POPS:NBD-PE lipid mixture was incubated with vesicles without methyl-α-cyclodextrin treatment as a control. In the absence of methyl-α-cyclodextrin treatment, control vesicles expressed limited fluorescence signals (**Figure 21A**). On the other hand, the lipid exchange with methyl-α-cyclodextrin treatment expressed strong fluorescence signals, which means that lipid exchange had occurred only in the presence of methyl-α-cyclodextrin treatment (**Figure 21B**).

Figure 21

(A) NBD expression in methyl-α-cyclodextrin treated and untreated GPMV vesicles. Scale bar=20 µm. ***(B)*** *Fluorescence intensity was measured based on the expression area per GPMV number using the NIS Elements software.* Samples *were imaged at 100X magnification and scale bar is 10 µm. The experiment was repeated three times and error bars represent the standard error and ** indicates $p < 0.01$.*

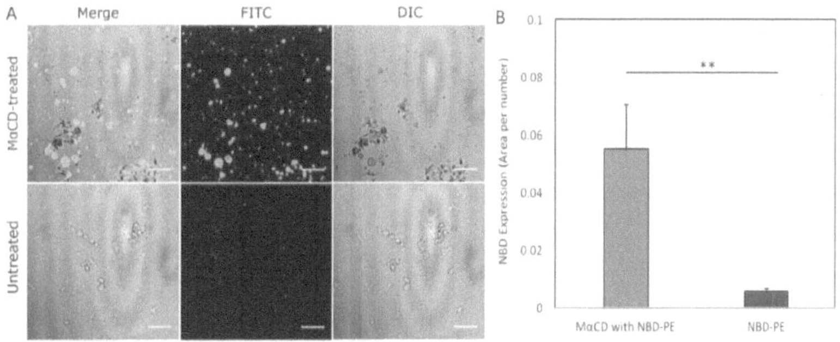

Examining the Role of Lipids in Membrane Integrity

Liposomal structures have been found to be more stable when their lipid composition is saturated.[182] Lian et al. have also confirmed that liposomes made up of unsaturated lipids were found to be much less stable than liposomes made up of saturated phospholipids.[183] In the presence or absence of POPS lipid exchange using the methyl-α-cyclodextrin treatment, the effect of single lipid exchange on the disruption of GPMV membranes was studied using the LDH membrane integrity kit. Results indicated that exchanging membrane lipids with POPS saturated lipids increased the stability of A549 cell membrane-derived vesicles (**Figure 22A**). Also, vesicles with more saturated lipids were disturbed less after exposure to silica nanoparticles (**Figure 22B**). As a result, POPS lipid exchange can repair the membrane damage after vesiculation rupture and increases the stability of GPMV vesicles in PBS and decreases the membrane disruption due to the silica nanoparticle exposure.

Figure 22

Stability characterization of membrane-based vesicles. ***(A)*** *Leakage study of lipid-exchanged GPMVs as measured by the release of lactate from the lumen of the vesicles in PBS, at 37° C, and pH of 7.4.* ***(B)*** *Comparison of intact and POPS lipid exchanged GPMV membranes derived from A549 cells. The experiment was repeated three times* *and error bars represent the standard deviation of at least three independent measurements.*

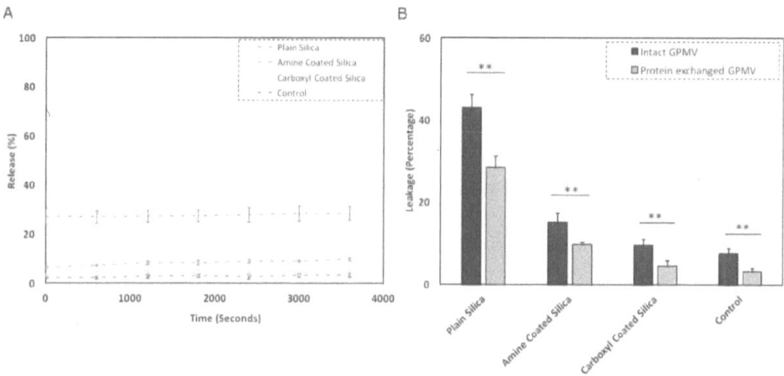

Examining the Role of Lipids in Nanoparticle Binding to the Membrane

The role of membrane lipids saturation in controlling the interaction between nanoparticles and plasma membranes was investigated using confocal fluorescent microscopy. The role of POPS saturated lipid in controlling nanoparticle-plasma membrane interactions was revealed by surface adsorption of nanoparticles onto GPMV membranes after exchanging membrane lipids with POPS by methyl-cyclodextrin treatment. Confocal images indicated a considerable fluctuation in membrane integrity of POPS exchanged vesicles after getting exposed to plain silica nanoparticles (**Figure 23A**). Also, the comparison of nanoparticle adsorption between the intact and POPS exchanged GPMV vesicles showed a significant reduction of surface adhesion after a single lipid exchange for plain nanoparticles (**Figure 23B**), which was predictable due to the repulsive force between the anionic headgroups of POPS and negatively charged silica nanoparticles especially the plain nanoparticles with the most negative surface zeta potential (**Table 1**).

Figure 23

Absorbance of plain, amine and carboxyl modified nanoparticles to the intact and lipid-exchanged GPMV vesicles derived of the A549 cells. ***(A)*** *Confocal microscopy images of POPS exchanged GPMVs.* ***(B)*** *Quantitative analysis based on the area of colocalization of two fluorescent probes per total cell membrane area measurement using NIS Elements. The experiment was repeated three times and error bar represent the standard deviation* *of the measurements.* Samples *were imaged at 100X magnification and scale bar is 5 μm.*

* *indicates* $p < 0.1$.

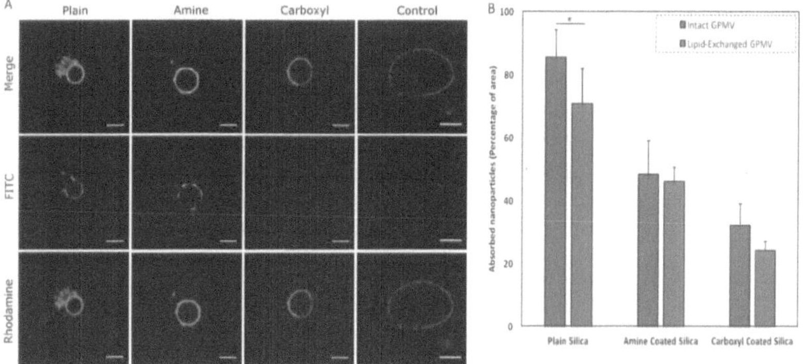

Flow cytometry was also used to further analyze the silica nanoparticle adsorption on the surface of the cell membrane-derived vesicles with and without the saturated lipid exchange. Different vesicle samples and silica nanoparticles were stained with the rhodamine-DOPE and FITC fluorescent probe, respectively. Flow cytometry results confirmed the previous experiment, indicating that POPS lipid exchange increased the negative charge of the GPMV membrane and induced more repulsive force against the negatively charged silica nanoparticles (**Figure 24**).

Figure 24

Absorbance of plain, amine and carboxyl modified nanoparticles to the surface of intact and POPS lipid exchanged GPMV vesicles derived of the A549 cells using the flow cytometry analysis. ***(A)*** *Flow cytometry dot plots showing vesicle and nanoparticle* *populations for: **(1)** Dot plot analysis of intact GPMVs vs. plain nanoparticles. **(2)** Dot plot analysis of intact GPMVs vs. amine-modified nanoparticles. **(3)** Dot plot analysis of intact GPMVs vs. carboxyl-modified nanoparticles. **(4)** Dot plot analysis of lipid exchanged GPMVs vs. plain nanoparticles. **(5)** Dot plot analysis of lipid exchanged GPMVs vs. amine-modified nanoparticles. **(6)** Dot plot analysis of lipid exchanged GPMVs vs. carboxyl-modified nanoparticles. **(B)** Intact and POPS exchanged vesicles and plain, amine-, and carboxyl-modified nanoparticles based on the positive population percentages (Q2 quadrant). The experiment was repeated three times and error bars represent the standard deviation of the measurements.*

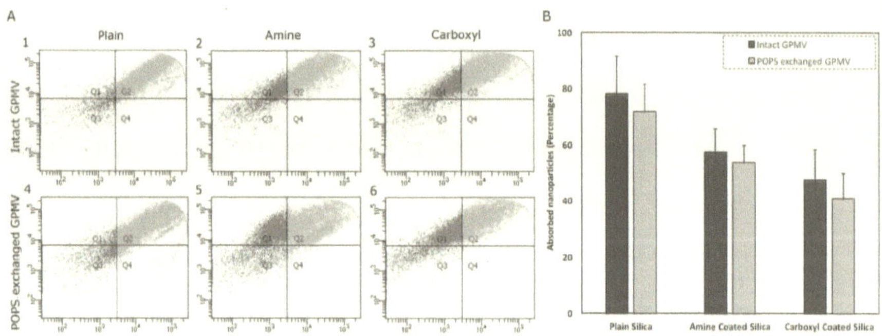

Fluorescence Anisotropy of Both Bilayers

DPH fluorescence anisotropy was used to investigate the influence of proteins and lipid saturation on the packing of membrane components in the biological vesicles. This fluorescent probe is capable of diving within the biological bilayer to assist in revealing the structural and dynamical properties of lipid bilayers. A significantly higher value of anisotropy was observed after POPS exogenous lipid exchange in the GPMV vesicles, indicating tight membrane packing of this vesicle after the addition of saturated lipids (**Figure 25**). On the other hand, the withdrawal of membrane proteins resulted in a significant reduction of membrane order in the protein-free vesicles.

Figure 25

DPH Anisotropy of cell membrane derived vesicles for lipid-exchanged, protein-free and intact GPMVs in PBS, at 37° C, and pH of 7.4. The experiment was repeated three times and error bar represent the standard deviation of the measurements. ***** *indicates p < 0. 00001.*

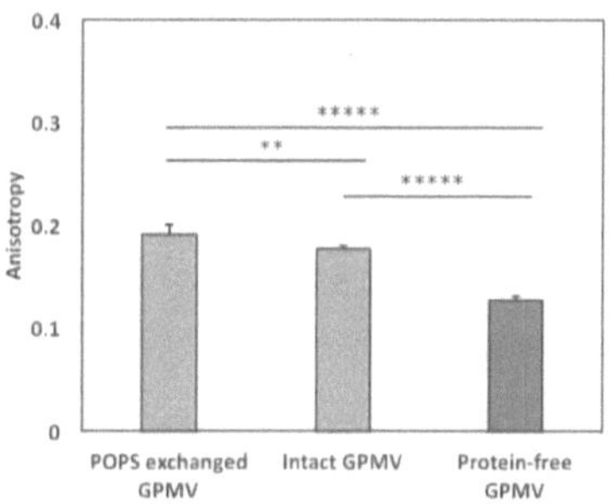

Fluorescence Anisotropy of External Bilayer

For the further examination of compositional effects on membrane packing of vesicles, fluorescence anisotropy was measured using the DPH after the addition of PMA in these membranes. As expected, vesicles containing the POPS saturated lipid showed a high value of TMA-DPH anisotropy, reflecting that the fluidity at the saturated lipid membrane surface is significantly lower than the anisotropy measured using the DPH, deeper in the membrane heart. In contrast, anisotropy of protein-free membrane did not change between the surface and depth of lipid bilayer, indicating a loose and equally distributed lipid packing in the absence of membrane compartmentalization by proteins (**Figure 26**).

Figure 26

TMA-DPH Anisotropy of cell membrane derived vesicles for lipid-exchanged, protein-free and intact GPMVs in PBS, at 37° C, and pH of 7.4. The experiment was repeated three times and error bar represent the standard deviation of the measurements. ***** *indicates p < 0. 00001.*

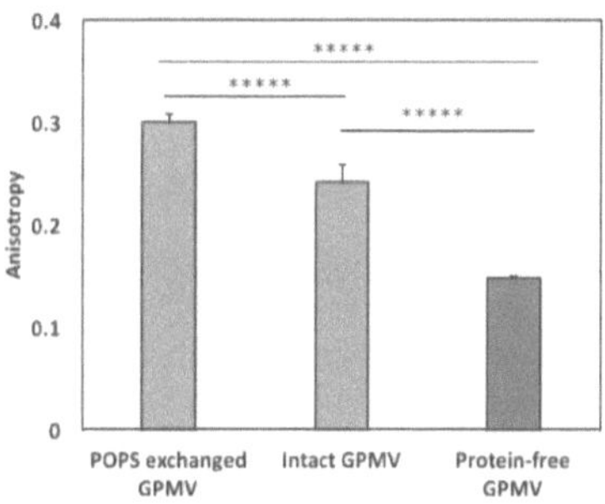

Discussion

Previous studies of nanoparticle-cell membrane interactions made it clear that the order of lipid phases and fluidity of plasma membrane has a crucial impact on the stability of membrane and surface adhesion of exogenous entities.[184] Numerous lipid bilayer membranes were developed to investigate the mechanism and factors influencing lipid order in the membrane. These lipid order studies confirm that the length and saturation of the phospholipids, as the most abundant membrane lipids, are key factors in the ability of membrane lipids to sit within different orders next to each other.[185] On the other hand, while it is possible to incorporate a few proteins within liposomal bilayers, this process has low efficiency and leads to patchy and close-packed random areas in the membrane.[166] Cell membrane-derived vesicles offer the closest approximation to the native cell membrane with the same order, orientation, and lipid and protein composition.

Ion channels and exchanger transmembrane proteins are responsible for the difference in the electrostatic potential of two sides of a membrane, known as the electrophysiological transmembrane potential.[186] The zeta potential is the term given to this surface potential defined by the charge of membrane components and the counterions in solution.[187] As a result, the function of transmembrane channels and other proteins is highly correlated to electrostatic zeta potentials. After withdrawing the membrane proteins, my zeta potential analysis revealed that the surface charge of GPMVs derived directly from A549 cells was less negative (**Table 2**). This trend is confirmed with a previous study by Surma et al. that suggests a high negative charge zeta potential was measured after incorporating proteins within the liposomal system.[188]

Cell membranes contain hundreds of different proteins, and they constantly interact with other membrane compounds in the biological bilayer to preserve lipid packaging, fluidity and permeability, charge, and overall integrity of cell membranes.[165] Membrane proteins have been shown to increase rigidity, mechanical strength, and stability while decreasing the fluidity of the lipid bilayer in plasma membranes.[189] However, our leakage study showed a higher release rate for cell membrane-derived vesicles that contain proteins compared to the protein-free GPMV vesicles (**Figure 18**). This unexpected result can be explained using the mechanism that vesiculation taken placed. Here, the GPMV vesicle isolation was utilized by chemical induction of cells and the rupture of blebs away from the plasma membrane. These ruptured patches are stable pores formed during the chemically-induced rupture of vesicles from cells.[58] My release study experiment verified several previously reported topography studies of GPMV membranes;[58,179] and made it clear that ruptured GPMV patches can significantly increase the leakiness of these membranes (**Figure 18**). Overall, stability results indicate that regardless of all the mechanical support that membrane proteins offer within the lipid bilayers, open pores of patchy GPMV membranes leak at a higher level than the uniform protein-free membranes.

Melby et al. have proven that the addition of membrane proteins to the structure of lipid bilayers can facilitate nanoparticle adhesion to the surface of the liposomes.[190] Proteins are especially important in the adsorption of negative nanoparticles due to mitigation of the repulsive force between the negatively charged cell membrane and nanoparticles.[172] As was expected based on previous work,[180] I quantified a higher level of nanoparticle-cell membrane association in the presence of membrane proteins (**Figure 19** and **20**). Therefore, proteins are the key element in the membrane, influencing almost all the cellular properties, including the shape, charge, stability, and communication with exogenous nanoparticles.

Fatty acid based lipids and proteins are two major components of the plasma membrane. The length and unsaturation level of acyl chains are two essential factors in membrane lipids, critical for the final charge, order, and orientation of the plasma membrane.[191] POPS has a negatively charged headgroup with one saturated and one monounsaturated acyl chain at carbon nine and 7.4 pH.[192] As was expected, the replacement of exogenous lipid with POPS increased the total negative charge of vesicles

(**Table 3**). POPS phospholipids play an important role in cell signaling, protein compartmentalization, and membrane organization as one of the most common negatively charged lipids in the cell membrane. Also, X-ray diffraction experiments by Khondker et al. showed liposomes formed from POPS have highly-oriented lipid bilayers.[193] Due to all of the structural benefits, POPS was selected for single lipid exchange in this study using the already established lipid exchange method by Li et al., and the exchange was confirmed using the fluorescent probe (**Figure 21**).[170]

The highly ordered POPS exchanged GPMV vesicles showed less leakage than intact GPMVs (**Figure 22**), which was predicted based on the study by Alhakamy et al., which reported an increase in the surface pressure after the addition of anionic POPS phospholipid compared to the other zwitterionic or less charged phospholipids.[194] Moreover, the POPS lipid exchanged GPMV membranes showed less surface adhesion than intact GPMVs for negatively charged nanoparticles (**Figure 22** and **23**), which was predictable due to the excessive repulsive force between the anionic headgroups of POPS and negatively charged silica nanoparticles. Also, less release was observed in the control group of lipid exchanged GPMVs than the unexchanged group, which I propose can be explained by the potential repairing ability of lipid-loaded Methyl-α-cyclodextrin in membrane pores.

Liu et al. showed that the addition of POPS in the liposomal structures influenced the total charge, stability, and ability of other compounds to pack against one another, thereby affecting the fluidity of the membrane.[195] My anisotropy studies also confirmed this finding, indicating the positive effect of POPS amphipathic lipid in enhancing the rigidity and order of membrane structures (**Figure 25**). The surface rigidity of POPS lipid exchanged vesicles showed a higher value using the TMA-DPH anisotropy, reflecting that the fluidity at the outer bilayer in which the lipid exchange took place is significantly higher than DPH anisotropy (**Figure 26**); this observation was expected because the DPH probe has proved to dive deeper in the heart of GPMV membranes.[176]

Altogether, the current work indicates that the presence of membrane protein and anionic, semi-saturated lipids within the GPMV vesicles significantly enhance the physicochemical properties of cell membrane-derived vesicles. Higher charge, stability, rigidness, degree of lipid and protein order, and nanoparticle adsorption are some of these benefits that make the lipid exchanged protein-containing cell membrane-derived vesicles a great candidate for drug/nanoparticle delivery and membrane model studies.

Chapter 5: Conclusions and Future Work

Nanoparticles are currently being widely studied for different therapeutic and diagnostic applications. However, solid nanoparticles have been associated with various toxicity-related issues, with one particular issue being their toxicity induced by damage to the cell plasma membrane. It is thus generally recognized that more research is needed to increase the targeting efficiency, reduce the toxicity, and elucidate the mechanisms by which drug delivery vehicles induce toxicity. In the attempt to solve this problem, recent investigations have focused on two goals (1) introducing different membrane mimicking cargos that mimic the bilayer membrane of the cell and (2) coating the toxic entities with a biocompatible layer in order to reduce the systemic toxicity.

The fundamental principle of these efforts is based on improving the efficiency of the existing techniques or creating brand-new solutions. Many of these biomedical nanotechnology movements were successfully evolved into advanced diagnostic and therapeutic approaches, which paved the road for a considerable improvement of healthcare quality and patient safety. However, despite all the improvements, many challenges still remain. Acute systemic toxicity, due to the drug interacting with healthy cells, is one of these major challenges that is an unacceptable side effect.

The concept of drug delivery systems has been introduced first as "the magical bullet" by Paul Elrich in 1909, with the purpose of dissolving the central systemic toxicity issue. Developing non-invasive and highly targeted platforms has been a challenge and a goal for many decades. From then till now, thousands of drug delivery systems have been developed and evolved with the advances in material and biochemistry sciences. Nevertheless, despite recent delivery nanostructure advances, continued researches are required to discover the efficient approaches for revolutionizing the current hurdles of systemic delivery systems.

Several different types of hard, soft, natural, and artificial vesicles have been developed, with and without targeting agents, to improve the targeting accuracy, binding capacity, cellular uptake, and internalization levels of therapeutic agents in diseased cells while minimizing toxicity to healthy normal cells. The use of drug delivery systems is a desirable approach to successfully fulfill these delivery-related factors and facilitate drug accumulation at the intended site of action. However, several challenges remain to be addressed before delivery systems can be adopted successfully in clinical trials for patients.

First, there is still limited understanding of the complex delivery pharmacokinetic properties and their correlated pharmacodynamic effects at the desired action sites. In other terms, there is a lack of sufficient knowledge about how physiologically relevant conditions, such as the hydrodynamic conditions of blood flow, can affect the recognition, adhesion, and internalization of nanoparticles by target cells. Nevertheless, there is still very limited understanding of the absorption and distribution of different carriers in the bloodstream. The circulatory system is one of the main transportation systems to deliver therapeutics into diverse organs and selective targets. Therefore, understanding the *in vivo* behaviors of each pharmacological route is very vital for the translation of laboratory *in vitro* static to physciologic *in vivo* dynamic conditions. Consequently, further research is needed to identify the effect of blood flow shear stress and other transport effects in nanoparticle-drug transportation within the circulatory system.

Additionally, in order to get better control of the delivery process, new coatings are required to accommodate targeting motifs embedded within their membrane mimicking shells. Major advances have been made during the past decade in the field of targeted drug delivery. Newly commercialized targeted therapies have revolutionized the traditional aggressive therapeutic approaches. Yet, not many targeted treatments are presently available at the clinical level. Targeted medication, which is currently available, may not be the right option for every patient. While it can seem straightforward, targeted therapy is complex, and it may not always function if the unhealthy area does not display a proper amount of molecular targeting motifs, therapeutic carrier adhesion, or significant drug efficiency. Therefore, further development and translation of efficient targeting techniques are necessary to facilitate nanoparticle/drug accumulation in the desired cellular compartments.

Furthermore, pharmaceutical technology scientists are still struggling to engineer an advanced coating in order to avoid immune system recognition. The ultimate goal is to produce an ideal coating capable of evading immunological responses from macrophage cells. Much effort has been centered lately on developing a less invasive coating with a high level of similarities to the native cell membranes. In my dissertation, I have first utilized liposomes as a delivery cargo. Liposomes are semi-spherical-shaped vesicles that closely resemble the bilayer structure of plasma cell membranes. Additionally, I applied liposomes as the targeted drug delivery vehicles to the specific site of VCAM1 overexpression in atherosclerosis. My studies indicate that anti-VCAM1 functionalized system is capable of targeting and binding to epithelial cells that overexpress vascular cell adhesion molecule-1 (VCAM1). I have shown that this functionalized liposomal system can target the cells of interest under both static and physiologically relevant blood flow conditions.

Regardless of their bilayer assembly, proteins are not incorporated into the matrix of liposomes. While it is possible to incorporate one or a few proteins within the lipid-made structures, mimicking the exact composition, distribution, and orientation of proteins in the native structure of the plasma membrane is difficult. For all these reasons, I have then focused on developing a novel cell-derived drug loading technique to incorporate all membrane lipids and proteins in the final delivery cargo. Therefore, in the next step, I have utilized giant plasma membrane vesicles (GPMVs) to construct a cell membrane-derived and safe delivery platform that prevents the time-consuming steps of making protein-functionalized liposomes.

Additionally, I have introduced a novel loading technique to encapsulate drugs or drug-loaded therapeutic particles inside the cell membrane-derived vesicles. My data showed successful encapsulation of silica nanoparticles inside GPMVs isolated from A549 cells. I showed that nanoparticle encapsulation did not considerably change lipid/protein composition and physical properties of such GPMV-based core-shell structures. My further investigation also indicated a significant reduction in exogenously-induced toxicity after encapsulating nanotoxins inside the GPMVs, before exposing them to the recipient cells.

Then, I have focused on understanding the mechanism underlying the disruptive effects of nanoparticles on the cell membrane. Nanoparticle toxicity still remains an issue with many drug delivery vehicles, and there is a need to better understand the mechanisms of nanotoxicity. I used GPMVs to examine the toxicity level of different types of solid nanoparticles to the cell plasma membrane. My data indicated that surface engineering and the chemical composition of lipid membranes control their interactions with cells and exogenous materials.

In my latest work, I have introduced a novel repair technique to reconstruct pores that were formed during the GPMV vesiculation process. Endogenous lipid exchange in the living cells using the methyl-α-cyclodextrin was just introduced in the past decade (2010s). However, to the best of my knowledge, this is for the first time demonstrating a new repair application for methyl-α-cyclodextrin catalyzed treatment in vesicles derived directly from the living cells. My studies have shown a significant improvement in the stability and fluidity of GPMV vesicles after the saturated glycerophospholipid exchange compared to the non-exchanged GPMVs, before and after exposing them to different types of toxic nanoparticles.

Together, my research indicates that functionalization of delivery systems using the anti-VCAM1 antibodies improves the localization of these carriers on the inflamed endothelium. Charge and saturation of membrane lipids and selective incorporation of proteins are the key factors in nanoparticle binding, vesicle stability, and exogenously-induced disruption of cell membrane-derived delivery cargos. GPMV vesicles are capable of encapsulating different drugs and nanoparticles using the newly introduced parental uptake technique. Methyl-α-cyclodextrin catalyzed treatment is effectively capable of repairing the open pores formed during vesicle ruptures. Thus, careful and selective targeting of inflamed endothelium occurs using the VCAM1 functionalization of delivery systems; the parental loading technique results in cytosol compound transfer and drug loading within the GPMV delivery vesicles; and the incorporation of proteins and addition of highly charged and saturation lipids exchange can optimize the physicochemical properties of cell membrane-derived vesicles, which could lead to introducing a highly noninvasive and effective cell membrane-based drug delivery systems.

References

1. Loghin, M. E. & Kleiman, A. Medication-Induced neurotoxicity in critically Ill cancer PATIENTS. *Oncologic Critical Care* 319–334 (2020).

2. Wong, G., Sime, F. B., Lipman, J. & Roberts, J. A. How do we use therapeutic drug monitoring to improve outcomes from severe infections in critically ill patients? *BMC infectious diseases* **14**, 1–11 (2014).

3. Tiwari, G. *et al.* Drug delivery systems: An updated review. *International journal of pharmaceutical investigation* **2**, 2 (2012).

4. Yun, Y. H., Lee, B. K. & Park, K. Controlled drug delivery: Historical perspective for the next generation. *Journal of Controlled Release* **219**, 2–7 (2015).

5. Li, C. *et al.* Recent progress in drug delivery. *Acta Pharmaceutica Sinica B* **9**, 1145–1162 (2019).

6. Banerjee, R. Liposomes: applications in medicine. *Journal of Biomaterials applications* **16**, 3–21 (2001).

7. Mijajlovic, M., Wright, D., Zivkovic, V., Bi, J. X. & Biggs, M. J. Microfluidic hydrodynamic focusing based synthesis of POPC liposomes for model biological systems. *Colloids and surfaces B: biointerfaces* **104**, 276–281 (2013).

8. Bozzuto, G. & Molinari, A. Liposomes as nanomedical devices. *International journal of nanomedicine* **10**, 975 (2015).

9. Bangham, A. D., Hill, M. W. & Miller, N. G. A. Preparation and use of liposomes as models of biological membranes. in *Methods in membrane biology* 1–68 (Springer, 1974).

10. Pinheiro, M., Magalhães, J. & Reis, S. Antibiotic interactions using liposomes as model lipid membranes. *Chemistry and physics of lipids* **222**, 36–46 (2019).

11. Kimelberg, H. K. Protein-liposome interactions and their relevance to the structure and function of cell membranes. *Molecular and cellular biochemistry* **10**, 171–190 (1976).

12. Parmar, M. M., Edwards, K. & Madden, T. D. Incorporation of bacterial membrane proteins into liposomes: factors influencing protein reconstitution. *Biochimica et Biophysica Acta (BBA)-Biomembranes* **1421**, 77–90 (1999).

13. Angrand, M., Briolay, A., Ronzon, F. & Roux, B. Detergent-mediated reconstitution of a glycosyl-phosphatidylinositol-protein into liposomes. *European journal of biochemistry* **250**, 168–176 (1997).

14. Rigaud, J.-L., Pitard, B. & Levy, D. Reconstitution of membrane proteins into liposomes: application to energy-transducing membrane proteins. *Biochimica et Biophysica Acta (BBA)-Bioenergetics* **1231**, 223–246 (1995).

15. Levental, K. R. & Levental, I. Giant plasma membrane vesicles: models for understanding membrane organization. in *Current topics in membranes* vol. 75 25–57 (Elsevier, 2015).

16. Jokhadar, Š. Z. *et al.* GPMVs in variable physiological conditions: could they be used for therapy delivery? *BMC biophysics* **11**, 1 (2018).

17. Patra, J. K. *et al.* Nano based drug delivery systems: recent developments and future prospects. *Journal of nanobiotechnology* **16**, 71 (2018).

18. De Villiers, M. M., Aramwit, P. & Kwon, G. S. *Nanotechnology in drug delivery.*

(Springer Science & Business Media, 2008).

19. Dhoot, N. O. & Wheatley, M. A. Microencapsulated liposomes in controlled drug delivery: strategies to modulate drug release and eliminate the burst effect. *Journal of pharmaceutical sciences* **92**, 679–689 (2003).

20. Xia, S. *et al.* Modulating effect of lipid bilayer–carotenoid interactions on the property of liposome encapsulation. *Colloids and Surfaces B: Biointerfaces* **128**, 172–180 (2015).

21. Pagano, R. E. & Weinstein, J. N. Interactions of liposomes with mammalian cells. *Annual review of biophysics and bioengineering* **7**, 435–468 (1978).

22. Straubinger, R. M., Hong, K., Friend, D. S. & Papahadjopoulos, D. Endocytosis of liposomes and intracellular fate of encapsulated molecules: encounter with a low pH compartment after internalization in coated vesicles. *Cell* **32**, 1069–1079 (1983).

23. Letchford, K. & Burt, H. A review of the formation and classification of amphiphilic block copolymer nanoparticulate structures: micelles, nanospheres, nanocapsules and polymersomes. *European journal of pharmaceutics and biopharmaceutics* **65**, 259–269 (2007).

24. Blume, G. & Cevc, G. Liposomes for the sustained drug release in vivo. *Biochimica et Biophysica Acta (BBA)-Biomembranes* **1029**, 91–97 (1990).

25. Sanchez, L., Yi, Y. & Yu, Y. Effect of partial PEGylation on particle uptake by macrophages. *Nanoscale* **9**, 288–297 (2017).

26. Suk, J. S., Xu, Q., Kim, N., Hanes, J. & Ensign, L. M. PEGylation as a strategy for improving nanoparticle-based drug and gene delivery. *Advanced drug delivery*

reviews **99**, 28–51 (2016).

27. Libby, P., Ridker, P. M. & Maseri, A. Inflammation and atherosclerosis. *Circulation* **105**, 1135–1143 (2002).

28. Wierer, M. *et al.* Compartment-resolved proteomic analysis of mouse aorta during atherosclerotic plaque formation reveals osteoclast-specific protein expression. *Molecular & Cellular Proteomics* **17**, 321–334 (2018).

29. Naghavi, M. *et al.* From vulnerable plaque to vulnerable patient—part III: executive summary of the Screening for Heart Attack Prevention and Education (SHAPE) Task Force report. *The American journal of cardiology* **98**, 2–15 (2006).

30. Trialists, C. T. Efficacy of cholesterol-lowering therapy in 18 686 people with diabetes in 14 randomised trials of statins: a meta-analysis. *The Lancet* **371**, 117–125 (2008).

31. Layek, B. & Singh, J. *Editorial of special issue "Surface-functionalized nanoparticles as drug carriers"*. (Multidisciplinary Digital Publishing Institute, 2019).

32. Winter, P. M. *et al.* Molecular imaging of angiogenesis in early-stage atherosclerosis with αvβ3-integrin–targeted nanoparticles. *Circulation* **108**, 2270–2274 (2003).

33. Da Silva-Candal, A. *et al.* Shape effect in active targeting of nanoparticles to inflamed cerebral endothelium under static and flow conditions. *Journal of Controlled Release* **309**, 94–105 (2019).

34. Deosarkar, S. P. *et al.* Polymeric particles conjugated with a ligand to VCAM-1 exhibit selective, avid, and focal adhesion to sites of atherosclerosis. *Biotechnology*

and bioengineering **101**, 400–407 (2008).

35. Davies, M. J. *et al.* The expression of the adhesion molecules ICAM-1, VCAM-1, PECAM, and E-selectin in human atherosclerosis. *The Journal of pathology* **171**, 223–229 (1993).

36. Rubio-Guerra, A. F. *et al.* Correlation between the levels of circulating adhesion molecules and atherosclerosis in hypertensive type-2 diabetic patients. *Clinical and experimental hypertension* **32**, 308–310 (2010).

37. Sun, T. *et al.* Targeted delivery of anti-miR-712 by VCAM1-binding Au nanospheres for atherosclerosis therapy. *ChemNanoMat* **2**, 400–406 (2016).

38. Mlinar, L. B., Chung, E. J., Wonder, E. A. & Tirrell, M. Active targeting of early and mid-stage atherosclerotic plaques using self-assembled peptide amphiphile micelles. *Biomaterials* **35**, 8678–8686 (2014).

39. Pan, H. *et al.* Programmable nanoparticle functionalization for in vivo targeting. *The FASEB Journal* **27**, 255–264 (2013).

40. Li, Y.-S. J., Haga, J. H. & Chien, S. Molecular basis of the effects of shear stress on vascular endothelial cells. *Journal of biomechanics* **38**, 1949–1971 (2005).

41. Galbraith, C. G., Skalak, R. & Chien, S. Shear stress induces spatial reorganization of the endothelial cell cytoskeleton. *Cell motility and the cytoskeleton* **40**, 317–330 (1998).

42. Ng, C. P. & Pun, S. H. A perfusable 3D cell–matrix tissue culture chamber for in situ evaluation of nanoparticle vehicle penetration and transport. *Biotechnology and bioengineering* **99**, 1490–1501 (2008).

43. Date, A. A., Joshi, M. D. & Patravale, V. B. Parasitic diseases: liposomes and polymeric nanoparticles versus lipid nanoparticles. *Advanced drug delivery reviews* **59**, 505–521 (2007).

44. Fang, R. H., Luk, B. T., Hu, C.-M. J. & Zhang, L. Engineered nanoparticles mimicking cell membranes for toxin neutralization. *Advanced drug delivery reviews* **90**, 69–80 (2015).

45. Zhang, K., Fang, H., Chen, Z., Taylor, J.-S. A. & Wooley, K. L. Shape effects of nanoparticles conjugated with cell-penetrating peptides (HIV Tat PTD) on CHO cell uptake. *Bioconjugate chemistry* **19**, 1880–1887 (2008).

46. Fang, R. H., Jiang, Y., Fang, J. C. & Zhang, L. Cell membrane-derived nanomaterials for biomedical applications. *Biomaterials* **128**, 69–83 (2017).

47. Schauer, R. Sialic acids as regulators of molecular and cellular interactions. *Current opinion in structural biology* **19**, 507–514 (2009).

48. Zerial, M. & McBride, H. Rab proteins as membrane organizers. *Nature reviews Molecular cell biology* **2**, 107–117 (2001).

49. Shaffer, K. L., Sharma, A., Snapp, E. L. & Hegde, R. S. Regulation of protein compartmentalization expands the diversity of protein function. *Developmental cell* **9**, 545–554 (2005).

50. Jahn, R. & Fasshauer, D. Molecular machines governing exocytosis of synaptic vesicles. *Nature* **490**, 201–207 (2012).

51. Maza, N. A., Schiesser, W. E. & Calvert, P. D. An intrinsic compartmentalization code for peripheral membrane proteins in photoreceptor neurons. *Journal of Cell*

Biology **218**, 3753–3772 (2019).

52. Sezgin, E. *et al.* Elucidating membrane structure and protein behavior using giant plasma membrane vesicles. *Nature protocols* 7, 1042 (2012).

53. Steinkühler, J., Sezgin, E., Urbančič, I., Eggeling, C. & Dimova, R. Mechanical properties of plasma membrane vesicles correlate with lipid order, viscosity and cell density. *Communications biology* **2**, 1–8 (2019).

54. Czogalla, A., Grzybek, M., Jones, W. & Coskun, Ü. Validity and applicability of membrane model systems for studying interactions of peripheral membrane proteins with lipids. *Biochimica et Biophysica Acta (BBA)-Molecular and Cell Biology of Lipids* **1841**, 1049–1059 (2014).

55. Sun, D. *et al.* A novel nanoparticle drug delivery system: the anti-inflammatory activity of curcumin is enhanced when encapsulated in exosomes. *Molecular Therapy* **18**, 1606–1614 (2010).

56. Säälik, P. *et al.* Penetration without cells: membrane translocation of cell-penetrating peptides in the model giant plasma membrane vesicles. *Journal of controlled release* **153**, 117–125 (2011).

57. Pae, J. *et al.* Translocation of cell-penetrating peptides across the plasma membrane is controlled by cholesterol and microenvironment created by membranous proteins. *Journal of Controlled Release* **192**, 103–113 (2014).

58. Skinkle, A. D., Levental, K. R. & Levental, I. Cell-derived plasma membrane vesicles are permeable to hydrophilic macromolecules. *Biophysical Journal* (2020).

59. Creixell, M., Bohorquez, A. C., Torres-Lugo, M. & Rinaldi, C. EGFR-targeted

magnetic nanoparticle heaters kill cancer cells without a perceptible temperature rise. *ACS nano* **5**, 7124–7129 (2011).

60. Premnath, P., Tan, B. & Venkatakrishnan, K. Engineering functionalized multi-phased silicon/silicon oxide nano-biomaterials to passivate the aggressive proliferation of cancer. *Scientific reports* **5**, 1–12 (2015).

61. Sandler, S. E., Fellows, B. & Mefford, O. T. *Best practices for characterization of magnetic nanoparticles for biomedical applications*. (ACS Publications, 2019).

62. Li, L. *et al.* Superparamagnetic iron oxide nanoparticles as MRI contrast agents for non-invasive stem cell labeling and tracking. *Theranostics* **3**, 595 (2013).

63. Manke, A., Wang, L. & Rojanasakul, Y. Mechanisms of nanoparticle-induced oxidative stress and toxicity. *BioMed research international* **2013**, (2013).

64. Borm, P. J. & Kreyling, W. Toxicological hazards of inhaled nanoparticles—potential implications for drug delivery. *Journal of nanoscience and nanotechnology* **4**, 521–531 (2004).

65. Sardari, R. R. R. *et al.* Toxicological effects of silver nanoparticles in rats. *Afr J Microbiol Res* **6**, 5587–5593 (2012).

66. Lin, W., Huang, Y., Zhou, X.-D. & Ma, Y. In vitro toxicity of silica nanoparticles in human lung cancer cells. *Toxicology and applied pharmacology* **217**, 252–259 (2006).

67. Eom, H.-J. & Choi, J. Oxidative stress of silica nanoparticles in human bronchial epithelial cell, Beas-2B. *Toxicology in Vitro* **23**, 1326–1332 (2009).

68. Qhobosheane, M., Santra, S., Zhang, P. & Tan, W. Biochemically functionalized

silica nanoparticles. *Analyst* **126**, 1274–1278 (2001).

69. Kim, I.-Y., Joachim, E., Choi, H. & Kim, K. Toxicity of silica nanoparticles depends on size, dose, and cell type. *Nanomedicine: Nanotechnology, Biology and Medicine* **11**, 1407–1416 (2015).

70. Yu, T., Malugin, A. & Ghandehari, H. Impact of silica nanoparticle design on cellular toxicity and hemolytic activity. *ACS nano* **5**, 5717–5728 (2011).

71. Jin, Y., Kannan, S., Wu, M. & Zhao, J. X. Toxicity of luminescent silica nanoparticles to living cells. *Chemical research in toxicology* **20**, 1126–1133 (2007).

72. Yin, N. *et al.* Silver nanoparticle exposure attenuates the viability of rat cerebellum granule cells through apoptosis coupled to oxidative stress. *Small* **9**, 1831–1841 (2013).

73. Arai, Y., Miyayama, T. & Hirano, S. Difference in the toxicity mechanism between ion and nanoparticle forms of silver in the mouse lung and in macrophages. *Toxicology* **328**, 84–92 (2015).

74. Cooper, G. M. & Hausman, R. E. The cell: a molecular approach. Sinauer Associates. *Sunderland, MA* (2000).

75. Van Meer, G., Voelker, D. R. & Feigenson, G. W. Membrane lipids: where they are and how they behave. *Nature reviews Molecular cell biology* **9**, 112–124 (2008).

76. Otterbach, B. & Stoffel, W. Acid sphingomyelinase-deficient mice mimic the neurovisceral form of human lysosomal storage disease (Niemann-Pick disease). *Cell* **81**, 1053–1061 (1995).

77. Lin, Q. & London, E. Preparation of artificial plasma membrane mimicking

vesicles with lipid asymmetry. *PloS one* **9**, (2014).

78. Farnoud, A. M., Toledo, A. M., Konopka, J. B., Del Poeta, M. & London, E. Raft-like membrane domains in pathogenic microorganisms. in *Current topics in membranes* vol. 75 233–268 (Elsevier, 2015).

79. Shinto, H., Fukasawa, T., Yoshisue, K., Tezuka, M. & Orita, M. Cell membrane disruption induced by amorphous silica nanoparticles in erythrocytes, lymphocytes, malignant melanocytes, and macrophages. *Advanced Powder Technology* **25**, 1872–1881 (2014).

80. Verma, A. & Stellacci, F. Effect of surface properties on nanoparticle–cell interactions. *small* **6**, 12–21 (2010).

81. Farhood, H., Serbina, N. & Huang, L. The role of dioleoyl phosphatidylethanolamine in cationic liposome mediated gene transfer. *Biochimica et Biophysica Acta (BBA)-Biomembranes* **1235**, 289–295 (1995).

82. Bobryshev, Y. V. Monocyte recruitment and foam cell formation in atherosclerosis. *Micron* **37**, 208–222 (2006).

83. Moore, K. J., Sheedy, F. J. & Fisher, E. A. Macrophages in atherosclerosis: a dynamic balance. *Nature Reviews Immunology* **13**, 709–721 (2013).

84. Doll, R. Efficacy of cholesterol-lowering therapy in 18 686 people with diabetes in 14 randomised trials of statins: a meta-analysis. *Lancet* **371**, 117–125 (2008).

85. Bakker-Arkema, R. G. *et al.* A brief review paper of the efficacy and safety of atorvastatin in early clinical trials. *Atherosclerosis* **131**, 17–23 (1997).

86. Herd, J. A., West, M. S., Ballantyne, C., Farmer, J. & Gotto Jr, A. M. Baseline

characteristics of subjects in the lipoprotein and coronary atherosclerosis study (LCAS) with fluvastatin. *The American journal of cardiology* **73**, D42–D49 (1994).

87. Yoo, S. P. *et al.* Gadolinium-functionalized peptide amphiphile micelles for multimodal imaging of atherosclerotic lesions. *ACS omega* **1**, 996–1003 (2016).

88. Winter, P. M. *et al.* Endothelial αvβ3 integrin–targeted fumagillin nanoparticles inhibit angiogenesis in atherosclerosis. *Arteriosclerosis, thrombosis, and vascular biology* **26**, 2103–2109 (2006).

89. Chen, W. *et al.* Incorporation of an apoE-derived lipopeptide in high-density lipoprotein MRI contrast agents for enhanced imaging of macrophages in atherosclerosis. *Contrast media & molecular imaging* **3**, 233–242 (2008).

90. Cao, Z. *et al.* Reversible cell-specific drug delivery with aptamer-functionalized liposomes. *Angewandte Chemie International Edition* **48**, 6494–6498 (2009).

91. Lee, W., Yang, E.-J., Ku, S.-K., Song, K.-S. & Bae, J.-S. Anti-inflammatory effects of oleanolic acid on LPS-induced inflammation in vitro and in vivo. *Inflammation* **36**, 94–102 (2013).

92. Khodabandehlou, K., Masehi-Lano, J. J., Poon, C., Wang, J. & Chung, E. J. Targeting cell adhesion molecules with nanoparticles using in vivo and flow-based in vitro models of atherosclerosis. *Experimental Biology and Medicine* **242**, 799–812 (2017).

93. OHSAWA, T., MIURA, H. & HARADA, K. Improvement of encapsulation efficiency of water-soluble drugs in liposomes formed by the freeze-thawing method. *Chemical and pharmaceutical bulletin* **33**, 3945–3952 (1985).

94. Adib, A. A. *et al.* Engineered silica nanoparticles interact differently with lipid monolayers compared to lipid bilayers. *Environmental Science: Nano* **5**, 289–303 (2018).

95. Bendas, G., Krause, A., Bakowsky, U., Vogel, J. & Rothe, U. Targetability of novel immunoliposomes prepared by a new antibody conjugation technique. *International journal of pharmaceutics* **181**, 79–93 (1999).

96. Galkina, E. & Ley, K. Immune and inflammatory mechanisms of atherosclerosis. *Annual review of immunology* **27**, (2009).

97. Abràmoff, M. D., Magalhães, P. J. & Ram, S. J. Image processing with ImageJ. *Biophotonics international* **11**, 36–42 (2004).

98. Shirure, V. S., Reynolds, N. M. & Burdick, M. M. Mac-2 binding protein is a novel E-selectin ligand expressed by breast cancer cells. *PloS one* **7**, (2012).

99. Malek, A. M., Alper, S. L. & Izumo, S. Hemodynamic shear stress and its role in atherosclerosis. *Jama* **282**, 2035–2042 (1999).

100. Wang, F. & Liu, J. Nanodiamond decorated liposomes as highly biocompatible delivery vehicles and a comparison with carbon nanotubes and graphene oxide. *Nanoscale* **5**, 12375–12382 (2013)

101. Abraham, S., Brahim, S., Ishihara, K. & Guiseppi-Elie, A. Molecularly engineered p (HEMA)-based hydrogels for implant biochip biocompatibility. *Biomaterials* **26**, 4767–4778 (2005).

102. Namiki, M. *et al.* Local overexpression of monocyte chemoattractant protein-1 at vessel wall induces infiltration of macrophages and formation of atherosclerotic lesion:

synergism with hypercholesterolemia. *Arteriosclerosis, thrombosis, and vascular biology* **22**, 115–120 (2002).

103. Elbahnasawy, M. A., Donius, L. R., Reinherz, E. L. & Kim, M. Co-delivery of a CD4 T cell helper epitope via covalent liposome attachment with a surface-arrayed B cell target antigen fosters higher affinity antibody responses. *Vaccine* **36**, 6191–6201 (2018).

104. Gosk, S., Moos, T., Gottstein, C. & Bendas, G. VCAM-1 directed immunoliposomes selectively target tumor vasculature in vivo. *Biochimica et Biophysica Acta (BBA)-Biomembranes* **1778**, 854–863 (2008).

105. Mamot, C. *et al.* Epidermal growth factor receptor–targeted immunoliposomes significantly enhance the efficacy of multiple anticancer drugs in vivo. *Cancer research* **65**, 11631–11638 (2005).

106. Cybulsky, M. I. *et al.* A major role for VCAM-1, but not ICAM-1, in early atherosclerosis. *The Journal of clinical investigation* **107**, 1255–1262 (2001).

107. Ackers, I. & Malgor, R. Interrelationship of canonical and non-canonical Wnt signalling pathways in chronic metabolic diseases. *Diabetes and Vascular Disease Research* **15**, 3–13 (2018).

108. Konstantopoulos, K. & McIntire, L. V. Effects of fluid dynamic forces on vascular cell adhesion. *The Journal of clinical investigation* **98**, 2661–2665 (1996).

109. Bhowmick, T., Berk, E., Cui, X., Muzykantov, V. R. & Muro, S. Effect of flow on endothelial endocytosis of nanocarriers targeted to ICAM-1. *Journal of controlled release* **157**, 485–492 (2012).

110. Gu, W. *et al.* ICAM-1 regulates macrophage polarization by suppressing MCP-1 expression via miR-124 upregulation. *Oncotarget* **8**, 111882 (2017).

111. Yoon, H. J., Moon, M. E., Park, H. S., Im, S. Y. & Kim, Y. H. Chitosan oligosaccharide (COS) inhibits LPS-induced inflammatory effects in RAW 264.7 macrophage cells. *Biochemical and biophysical research communications* **358**, 954–959 (2007).

112. Zhu, L. *et al.* Fast fixing and comprehensive identification to help improve real-time ligands discovery based on formaldehyde crosslinking, immunoprecipitation and SDS-PAGE separation. *Proteome science* **12**, 1–8 (2014).

113. Cheung, L. S.-L. & Konstantopoulos, K. An analytical model for determining two-dimensional receptor-ligand kinetics. *Biophysical journal* **100**, 2338–2346 (2011).

114. McCarty, O. J., Mousa, S. A., Bray, P. F. & Konstantopoulos, K. Immobilized platelets support human colon carcinoma cell tethering, rolling, and firm adhesion under dynamic flow conditions. *Blood, The Journal of the American Society of Hematology* **96**, 1789–1797 (2000).

115. Jung, J. J., Grayson, K. A., King, M. R. & Lamkin-Kennard, K. A. Isolating the influences of fluid dynamics on selectin-mediated particle rolling at venular junctional regions. *Microvascular research* **118**, 144–154 (2018).

116. Evans, E. & Kinoshita, K. Using force to probe single-molecule receptor–cytoskeletal anchoring beneath the surface of a living cell. *Methods in cell biology* **83**, 373–396 (2007).

117. Finger, E. B. *et al.* Adhesion through L-selectin requires a threshold

hydrodynamic shear. *Nature* **379**, 266–269 (1996).

118. Tan, J., Thomas, A. & Liu, Y. Influence of red blood cells on nanoparticle targeted delivery in microcirculation. *Soft matter* **8**, 1934–1946 (2012).

119. Kheradmandi, M., Ackers, I., Burdick, M. M., Malgor, R. & Farnoud, A. M. Targeting dysfunctional vascular endothelial cells using immuno liposomes under flow conditions. *Cellular and Molecular Bioengineering* **13**, 189–199 (2020).

120. Escribá, P. V. *et al.* Membranes: a meeting point for lipids, proteins and therapies. *Journal of cellular and molecular medicine* **12**, 829–875 (2008).

121. Kersten, G. F. & Crommelin, D. J. Liposomes and ISCOMS. *Vaccine* **21**, 915–920 (2003).

122. Karp, G. The structure and function of the plasma membrane. *Cell and molecular biology: concepts and experiments, 3rd edn. New York: John Wiley and Sons* 122–82 (2002).

123. Tan, S., Wu, T., Zhang, D. & Zhang, Z. Cell or cell membrane-based drug delivery systems. *Theranostics* **5**, 863 (2015).

124. Le, Q.-V., Lee, J., Lee, H., Shim, G. & Oh, Y.-K. Cell membrane-derived vesicles for delivery of therapeutic agents. *Acta Pharmaceutica Sinica B* (2021).

125. Fang, R. H., Kroll, A. V., Gao, W. & Zhang, L. Cell membrane coating nanotechnology. *Advanced materials* **30**, 1706759 (2018).

126. Cinti, C., Taranta, M., Naldi, I. & Grimaldi, S. Newly engineered magnetic erythrocytes for sustained and targeted delivery of anti-cancer therapeutic compounds. *PloS one* **6**, e17132 (2011).

127. Hamidi, M., Zarrin, A. H., Foroozesh, M., Zarei, N. & Mohammadi-Samani, S. Preparation and in vitro evaluation of carrier erythrocytes for RES-targeted delivery of interferon-alpha 2b. *International journal of pharmaceutics* **341**, 125–133 (2007).

128. Harisa, G. I., Ibrahim, M. F., Alanazi, F. & Shazly, G. A. Engineering erythrocytes as a novel carrier for the targeted delivery of the anticancer drug paclitaxel. *Saudi Pharmaceutical Journal* **22**, 223–230 (2014).

129. Mishra, P. R. & Jain, N. K. Folate conjugated doxorubicin-loaded membrane vesicles for improved cancer therapy. *Drug Delivery* **10**, 277–282 (2003).

130. Rossi, L. *et al.* Heterodimer-loaded erythrocytes as bioreactors for slow delivery of the antiviral drug azidothymidine and the antimycobacterial drug ethambutol. *AIDS research and human retroviruses* **15**, 345–353 (1999).

131. Chen, Z. *et al.* Cancer cell membrane–biomimetic nanoparticles for homologous-targeting dual-modal imaging and photothermal therapy. *ACS nano* **10**, 10049–10057 (2016).

132. Ran, L. *et al.* Erythrocyte membrane-camouflaged nanoworms with on-demand antibiotic release for eradicating biofilms using near-infrared irradiation. *Bioactive materials* **6**, 2956–2968 (2021).

133. Lee, Y.-C. *et al.* Impact of detergents on membrane protein complex isolation. *Journal of proteome research* **17**, 348–358 (2018).

134. Guo, Y. Be cautious with crystal structures of membrane proteins or complexes prepared in detergents. *Crystals* **10**, 86 (2020).

135. Dang, X. T., Kavishka, J. M., Zhang, D. X., Pirisinu, M. & Le, M. T.

Extracellular vesicles as an efficient and versatile system for drug delivery. *Cells* **9**, 2191 (2020).

136. Dubavik, A. *et al.* Penetration of amphiphilic quantum dots through model and cellular plasma membranes. *Acs Nano* **6**, 2150–2156 (2012).

137. Bligh, E. G. Extraction of lipids in solution by the method of Bligh & Dyer. *Can J Biochem Physiol* **37**, 911–7 (1959).

138. Levchenko, T. S., Rammohan, R., Lukyanov, A. N., Whiteman, K. R. & Torchilin, V. P. Liposome clearance in mice: the effect of a separate and combined presence of surface charge and polymer coating. *International journal of pharmaceutics* **240**, 95–102 (2002).

139. Xu, J. *et al.* Integrated lipidomics and proteomics network analysis highlights lipid and immunity pathways associated with Alzheimer's disease. *Translational neurodegeneration* **9**, 1–15 (2020).

140. Eastlake, K. *et al.* Comparative proteomic analysis of normal and gliotic PVR retina and contribution of Müller glia to this profile. *Experimental eye research* **177**, 197–207 (2018).

141. Zhang, L. *et al.* Nanoparticles in medicine: therapeutic applications and developments. *Clinical pharmacology & therapeutics* **83**, 761–769 (2008).

142. Hung, H.-I. *et al.* PLGA nanoparticle encapsulation reduces toxicity while retaining the therapeutic efficacy of EtNBS-PDT in vitro. *Scientific reports* **6**, 1–13 (2016).

143. Sercombe, L. *et al.* Advances and challenges of liposome assisted drug delivery.

Frontiers in pharmacology **6**, 286 (2015).

144. Della Rocca, J., Huxford, R. C., Comstock-Duggan, E. & Lin, W. Polysilsesquioxane nanoparticles for targeted platin-based cancer chemotherapy by triggered release. *Angewandte Chemie International Edition* **50**, 10330–10334 (2011).

145. Belwal, V. K. & Singh, K. P. Nanosilica-supported liposome (protocells) as a drug vehicle for cancer therapy. *International journal of nanomedicine* **13**, 125 (2018).

146. Shagholani, H., Nikpay, A., Ghorbani, M. & Soltani, M. Synthesis and modification of crystalline SBA-15 nanowhiskers as a pH-sensitive metronidazole nanocarrier system. *International journal of pharmaceutics* **555**, 28–35 (2019).

147. Montazeri, M., Razzaghi-Abyaneh, M., Nasrollahi, S. A., Maibach, H. & Nafisi, S. Enhanced topical econazole antifungal efficacy by amine-functionalized silica nanoparticles. *Bulletin of Materials Science* **43**, 1–9 (2020).

148. Ahuja, S. & Dong, M. *Handbook of pharmaceutical analysis by HPLC*. (Elsevier, 2005).

149. Zhou, Y. *et al.* Integrated proteomics and lipidomics investigation of the mechanism underlying the neuroprotective effect of N-benzylhexadecanamide. *molecules* **23**, 2929 (2018).

150. Garnacho, C. Intracellular drug delivery: mechanisms for cell entry. *Current pharmaceutical design* **22**, 1210–1226 (2016).

151. Jedrzejczak-Silicka, M. & Mijowska, E. *General cytotoxicity and its application in nanomaterial analysis*. (IntechOpen London, UK, 2018).

152. Chong, C. S. *et al.* Enhancement of T helper type 1 immune responses against

hepatitis B virus core antigen by PLGA nanoparticle vaccine delivery. *Journal of controlled release* **102**, 85–99 (2005).

153. Fritsch-Decker, S. *et al.* Silica nanoparticles provoke cell death independent of p53 and BAX in human colon cancer cells. *Nanomaterials* **9**, 1172 (2019).

154. Vranic, S. *et al.* Impact of surface modification on cellular uptake and cytotoxicity of silica nanoparticles. (2020).

155. Bigdelou, P. Role of membrane asymmetry in nanoparticle-erythrocyte interactions. (Ohio University, 2020).

156. Andrews, D., Nann, T. & Lipson, R. H. *Comprehensive nanoscience and nanotechnology*. (Academic Press, 2019).

157. Capaldi, R. A. A dynamic model of cell membranes. *Scientific American* **230**, 26–33 (1974).

158. Uzman, A. *Molecular biology of the cell: Alberts, B., Johnson, A., Lewis, J., Raff, M., Roberts, K., and Walter, P.* (Wiley Online Library, 2003).

159. II, B., Pharm II, B. & II, B. Lipid chemistry.

160. Di Napoli, C. Label-free multiphoton microscopy of intracellular lipids using coherent anti-stokes raman scattering (CARS). (Cardiff University, 2014).

161. Poger, D. & Mark, A. E. A ring to rule them all: the effect of cyclopropane fatty acids on the fluidity of lipid bilayers. *The journal of physical chemistry B* **119**, 5487–5495 (2015).

162. Anderson, N. A., Richter, L. J., Stephenson, J. C. & Briggman, K. A. Characterization and control of lipid layer fluidity in hybrid bilayer membranes.

Journal of the American Chemical Society **129**, 2094–2100 (2007).

163. Leekumjorn, S. *et al.* The role of fatty acid unsaturation in minimizing biophysical changes on the structure and local effects of bilayer membranes. *Biochimica et Biophysica Acta (BBA)-Biomembranes* **1788**, 1508–1516 (2009).

164. Guidotti, G. Membrane proteins. *Annual review of biochemistry* **41**, 731–752 (1972).

165. Sankaram, M. B. & Marsh, D. Protein-lipid interactions with peripheral membrane proteins. in *New Comprehensive Biochemistry* vol. 25 127–162 (Elsevier, 1993).

166. Milhiet, P.-E. *et al.* High-resolution AFM of membrane proteins directly incorporated at high density in planar lipid bilayer. *Biophysical journal* **91**, 3268–3275 (2006).

167. Choi, M.-K. *et al.* Maintenance of membrane integrity and permeability depends on a patched-related protein in Caenorhabditis elegans. *Genetics* **202**, 1411–1420 (2016).

168. Cho, M.-H. *et al.* A bioluminescent cytotoxicity assay for assessment of membrane integrity using a proteolytic biomarker. *Toxicology in vitro* **22**, 1099–1106 (2008).

169. Kurtz-Chalot, A. *et al.* Adsorption at cell surface and cellular uptake of silica nanoparticles with different surface chemical functionalizations: impact on cytotoxicity. *Journal of nanoparticle research* **16**, 2738 (2014).

170. Li, G. *et al.* Efficient replacement of plasma membrane outer leaflet

phospholipids and sphingolipids in cells with exogenous lipids. *Proceedings of the National Academy of Sciences* **113**, 14025–14030 (2016).

171. Vahedi, A., Bigdelou, P. & Farnoud, A. M. Quantitative analysis of red blood cell membrane phospholipids and modulation of cell-macrophage interactions using cyclodextrins. *Scientific reports* **10**, 1–13 (2020).

172. Contini, C., Schneemilch, M., Gaisford, S. & Quirke, N. Nanoparticle–membrane interactions. *Journal of Experimental Nanoscience* **13**, 62–81 (2018).

173. de Planque, M. R., Aghdaei, S., Roose, T. & Morgan, H. Electrophysiological characterization of membrane disruption by nanoparticles. *ACS nano* **5**, 3599–3606 (2011).

174. Asghari Adib, A. Interactions of engineered silica nanoparticles with cell membrane models. (Ohio University, 2017).

175. Parasassi, T., Sapora, O., Giusti, A. M., De Stasio, G. & Ravagnan, G. Alterations in erythrocyte membrane lipids induced by low doses of ionizing radiation as revealed by 1, 6-diphenyl-1, 3, 5-hexatriene fluorescence lifetime. *International journal of radiation biology* **59**, 59–69 (1991).

176. Engel, L. W. & Prendergast, F. G. Values for and significance of order parameters and" cone angles" of fluorophore rotation in lipid bilayers. *Biochemistry* **20**, 7338–7345 (1981).

177. Honary, S. & Zahir, F. Effect of zeta potential on the properties of nano-drug delivery systems-a review (Part 1). *Tropical Journal of Pharmaceutical Research* **12**, 255–264 (2013).

178. Nishino, M. *et al.* Measurement and visualization of cell membrane surface charge in fixed cultured cells related with cell morphology. *Plos one* **15**, e0236373 (2020).

179. Chiang, P.-C., Tanady, K., Huang, L.-T. & Chao, L. Rupturing giant plasma membrane vesicles to form micron-sized supported cell plasma membranes with native transmembrane proteins. *Scientific reports* **7**, 1–8 (2017).

180. Chen, J. *et al.* Cationic nanoparticles induce nanoscale disruption in living cell plasma membranes. *The journal of physical chemistry B* **113**, 11179–11185 (2009).

181. Smith, M. C., Crist, R. M., Clogston, J. D. & McNeil, S. E. Zeta potential: a case study of cationic, anionic, and neutral liposomes. *Analytical and bioanalytical chemistry* **409**, 5779–5787 (2017).

182. Pietzyk, B. & Henschke, K. Degradation of phosphatidylcholine in liposomes containing carboplatin in dependence on composition and storage conditions. *International journal of pharmaceutics* **196**, 215–218 (2000).

183. Lian, T. & Ho, R. J. Trends and developments in liposome drug delivery systems. *Journal of pharmaceutical sciences* **90**, 667–680 (2001).

184. Olenick, L. L. *et al.* Lipid corona formation from nanoparticle interactions with bilayers. *Chem* **4**, 2709–2723 (2018).

185. Jones, A. E., Stolinski, M., Smith, R. D., Murphy, J. L. & Wootton, S. A. Effect of fatty acid chain length and saturation on the gastrointestinal handling and metabolic disposal of dietary fatty acids in women. *British Journal of Nutrition* **81**, 37–44 (1999).

186. Hodgkin, A. L. & Huxley, A. F. A quantitative description of membrane current and its application to conduction and excitation in nerve. *The Journal of physiology* **117**, 500–544 (1952).

187. Ma, Y., Poole, K., Goyette, J. & Gaus, K. Introducing membrane charge and membrane potential to T cell signaling. *Frontiers in immunology* **8**, 1513 (2017).

188. Surma, M. A., Szczepaniak, A. & Króliczewski, J. Comparative studies on detergent-assisted apocytochrome b 6 reconstitution into liposomal bilayers monitored by zetasizer instruments. *PloS one* **9**, e111341 (2014).

189. Dufourc, E. J. Sterols and membrane dynamics. *Journal of chemical biology* **1**, 63–77 (2008).

190. Melby, E. S. *et al.* Peripheral membrane proteins facilitate nanoparticle binding at lipid bilayer interfaces. *Langmuir* **34**, 10793–10805 (2018).

191. Manni, M. M. *et al.* Acyl chain asymmetry and polyunsaturation of brain phospholipids facilitate membrane vesiculation without leakage. *Elife* **7**, e34394 (2018).

192. Steinkopf, S. *et al.* The psychotropic drug olanzapine (Zyprexa®) increases the area of acid glycerophospholipid monolayers. *Biophysical chemistry* **134**, 39–46 (2008).

193. Khondker, A. *et al.* Membrane charge and lipid packing determine polymyxin-induced membrane damage. *Communications biology* **2**, 1–11 (2019).

194. Alhakamy, N. A., Elandaloussi, I., Ghazvini, S., Berkland, C. J. & Dhar, P. Effect of lipid headgroup charge and pH on the stability and membrane insertion potential of

calcium condensed gene complexes. *Langmuir* **31**, 4232–4245 (2015).

195. Liu, W., Wang, Z., Fu, L., Leblanc, R. M. & Yan, E. C. Lipid compositions modulate fluidity and stability of bilayers: characterization by surface pressure and sum frequency generation spectroscopy. *Langmuir* **29**, 15022–15031 (2013).

www.ingramcontent.com/pod-product-compliance
Lightning Source LLC
LaVergne TN
LVHW041107150826
845673LV00007B/1959

* 9 7 8 3 3 8 4 2 6 2 0 4 2 *